Medical Ethics: A Very Short Introduction

VERY SHORT INTRODUCTIONS are for anyone wanting a stimulating and accessible way into a new subject. They are written by experts, and have been translated into more than 45 different languages.

The series began in 1995, and now covers a wide variety of topics in every discipline. The VSI library currently contains over 550 volumes—a Very Short Introduction to everything from Psychology and Philosophy of Science to American History and Relativity—and continues to grow in every subject area.

Very Short Introductions available now:

For more information visit our website

www.oup.com/vsi/

Michael Dunn and Tony Hope

MEDICAL ETHICS

A Very Short Introduction

SECOND EDITION

OXFORD
UNIVERSITY PRESS

Great Clarendon Street, Oxford, OX2 6DP,
United Kingdom

Oxford University Press is a department of the University of Oxford.
It furthers the University's objective of excellence in research, scholarship,
and education by publishing worldwide. Oxford is a registered trade mark of
Oxford University Press in the UK and in certain other countries

First edition published in 2004
Second edition published in 2018

Impression: 1

Published in the United States of America by Oxford University Press
198 Madison Avenue, New York, NY 10016, United States of America

British Library Cataloguing in Publication Data
Data available

Library of Congress Control Number: 2018951235

ISBN 978-0-19-881560-0

Printed in Great Britain by
Ashford Colour Press Ltd, Gosport, Hampshire

This book is dedicated to our parents, Karen and Graham Dunn, and Marion and Ronald Hope, who inspired our love of reading and reasoning

Contents

Acknowledgements

TH would like to thank the following:

MTV Hart and the Royal Shakespeare Company who introduced me to philosophy.

Jonathan Glover whose philosophy tutorials are among the most stimulating intellectual experiences in my life.

Mike Gaze who supervised my PhD, and who showed me how experimental science and theoretical ideas could work together in creative tension.

Rosamond Rhodes and her colleagues at Mount Sinai Medical School in New York whose annual conference provided a critical but supportive forum for developing several of the ideas in this book.

Arthur Kuflik whose incisive comments, at all levels, on the draft manuscript of the first edition helped make many improvements.

My wife, Sally, my daughters Katy and Beth, and my son-in-law John Coull, for their support, discussions, and inspiration.

We would both like to thank: Tom Douglas, Josie Fielding, Helen Firth, and Mike Parker who gave valuable advice on aspects of this edition.

We have been stimulated and educated by discussions with many colleagues and friends, including: Nancy Berlinger, Jacqueline Chin, Isabel Clare, Nina Dunn, Kyle Edwards, Michael Gusmano, Tony Holland, Jonathan Ives, Camillia Kong, Gulamabbas Lakha, John McMillan, Leah Rand, Julian Savulescu, Mark Sheehan, Anne-Marie Slowther; Anne Stewart; Jacinta Tan; Mimi Zou, and further members of both The Ethox Centre and the Uehiro Centre.

We would like to thank all those at Oxford University Press who have helped to make this book possible and who have given their support and advice, and also an unknown reviewer.

Finally we would like to thank the staff of the Oxford Wine Café in Jericho, Oxford, who supplied us with space and drinks to enable our many discussions during the writing of this book.

List of illustrations

Chapter 1
On why medical ethics is exciting

Medical ethics will appeal to many temperaments: to the thinker and to the doer; to the philosopher and to the woman or man of action. It deals with some of the big moral questions: easing death and the morality of killing, for example. It takes us into the realm of politics. How should healthcare resources, necessarily limited, be distributed, and what should be the process for deciding? It is concerned with legal issues. Should it always be a crime for a doctor to practise euthanasia? When can a mentally ill person be treated against his will? And it leads us to the major world issue of the proper relationships between rich and poor countries.

Modern medical science creates new moral choices and challenges traditional views that we have of ourselves. Cloning has inspired many films and much concern. Detailed information about our genetic makeup and associated health risks can now be acquired with a sample of saliva and the touch of a screen. The possibility of editing our DNA is now a reality. Reproductive technologies raise the apparently abstract question of how we should think about the rights and interests of those who are yet to be born—and who may never exist. These questions lead us beyond medicine to consider our responsibilities towards the future of humankind.

Medical ethics ranges from the metaphysical to the mundanely practical. It is concerned not only with these large issues but also with everyday medical practice. Doctors get caught up in people's lives, and ordinary life is full of ethical tensions. An elderly woman with a degree of dementia suffers an acute life-threatening illness. Should she be treated in hospital with all the drugs and technology available; or should she be kept comfortable at home? The family cannot agree. There is nothing in this case likely to hit the headlines; but, as Auden's Old Masters knew, the ordinary is what is important to most of us, most of the time. In pursuing medical ethics we must be prepared to grapple with theory, allowing time for speculation and the use of the imagination. But we must also be ready to be practical: able to adopt a no-nonsense, down-to-earth approach that is sensitive to the ways each of us goes about our life.

Much emphasis during medical and nursing training is put on the importance of using scientific evidence correctly in clinical decision-making. Medical ethics endorses this feature of education, but recognizes that values, too, are a central feature of healthcare decisions. Just as the scientific and technical aspects of medicine need to be assessed and justified in terms of the evidence, so too must the ethical assumptions, values, and arguments be articulated and defended.

The philosopher and cultural historian, Isaiah Berlin, begins an essay on Tolstoy with the following words: 'There is a line among the fragments of the Greek poet Archilocus which says: "The fox knows many things, but the hedgehog knows one big thing".' Berlin goes on to suggest that, taken figuratively, this distinction between the fox and the hedgehog can mark 'one of the deepest differences which divide writers and thinkers, and, it may be, human beings in general' (see Figure 1).

The hedgehog represents those who relate everything to a central vision:

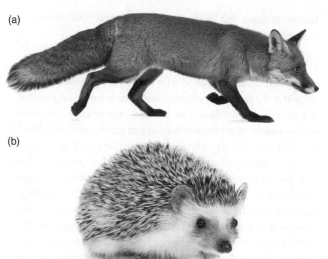

(a)

(b)

1. Are you a hedgehog or a fox?

one system less or more coherent or articulate, in terms of which they understand, think and feel—a single, universal, organizing principle in terms of which alone all that they are and say has significance.

The fox represents

those who pursue many ends, often unrelated and even contradictory, connected, if at all, only in some *de facto* way,…[who] lead lives, perform acts, and entertain ideas that are centrifugal rather than centripetal…seizing upon the essence of a vast variety of experiences…without…seeking to fit them into…any one unchanging, all-embracing,…unitary inner vision.

Berlin gives as examples of hedgehogs: Dante, Plato, Dostoevsky, Hegel, Proust, among others. He gives as examples of foxes: Shakespeare, Herodotus, Aristotle, Montaigne, and Joyce. Berlin

Why medical ethics is exciting

3

goes on to argue that Tolstoy was a fox by nature but believed in being a hedgehog.

Both of us are foxes, or at least aspire to be so. We admire the intellectual rigour of those who try to produce a unitary vision, but we prefer the rich, contradictory, and sometimes chaotic visions of Berlin's foxes. We do not, in this book, attempt to approach the various problems we discuss from one single moral theory. Nor do we give privileged position to any particular standpoint: doctor, nurse, physiotherapist, social worker, researcher, patient, or family member. Although this book is called *Medical Ethics*, its scope encompasses all aspects of treating, managing, and conducting research into illness and disease—activities that involve a wide range of health and care professionals working alongside each other. Equally, the book aims to highlight ethical issues that are not explicitly medical, arising as they do for those receiving care across all kinds of settings, such as hospitals, surgeries, nursing homes, and, indeed, patients' own homes.

Each chapter takes an ethical issue. We consider the various positions and, on occasion, we will argue for one particular ethical conclusion. We use whatever methods of argument seem to us to be the most relevant to making progress in addressing the difficult ethical decisions that healthcare professionals, and society, need to take.

On the distinctiveness of medical ethics

It is the role that argument plays that goes some way towards identifying the distinctiveness of medical ethics from related activities: medical law, political activism, and the social sciences relating to medicine.

Argument has a central place in medical law, as it does in medical ethics. But the foundation of the argument, and the role that the conclusions play, are different. In the case of law, the foundations

4

of the arguments are those principles set out in statutes, or that are either implied, or explicit, in previous legal judgements. In the case of ethics, however, the principles are not given—indeed much of the argument in ethics might be about what are the ethically right principles relevant to this situation, and why. Again, although the argument in both disciplines will be concerned with how to apply principles to specific situations, the law will be constrained in such application to similar situations in previous legal judgements. Ethics, while perhaps guided by previous applications, is never constrained. There is always a sceptical voice, sometimes in a shout, sometimes in *sotto voce*, which says: that might be what we thought before, but *were we right to do so?* In democratic societies laws are made by parliament (or similar legislative bodies) and through decisions in the courts. Both parliament and the courts, no doubt, wish to come to *ethically* correct decisions. So, ethics is primary: what is ethically correct should underpin medical law, but what is legally the case should not underpin ethics. In medical law this has been particularly evident. Many of the statutes and court decisions that are relevant to medical practice have been based on previous ethical analyses. The great Greek philosopher, Socrates, questioned the elite of society, demanding that they justify, through argument, their decisions and beliefs. He saw himself as a gadfly—disturbing the status quo, questioning the assumptions—in order to improve the moral basis of society. Medical ethics can, and should, act as a gadfly to medical law. There is always the question: is the law (ethically) right? And if it is not, that is a good reason for changing the law.

There is a further sense in which medical ethics is primary. Medical ethics is not only concerned with the question of whether a law is right, it is concerned also with the question of how and whether a medical situation ought to be governed, or regulated, by the law at all. Sometimes ethical considerations will lead to the conclusion that an issue ought to fall within the remit of the professional judgement of the individual practitioner, or within regulation by the professional bodies, but not by the law of the land.

The *role* of law is also very different from that of ethics. Society enforces laws, on healthcare professionals as on others, through punishment or compensation. In general, society demands that healthcare professionals follow the law. But there remains an ethical question for the professionals themselves: should they, in this situation, obey the law? In most situations the answer will be *yes*. Even if an individual believes the law to be ethically wrong, there is an ethical imperative that, as individuals, we respect society's laws, especially in a democracy. But there are many examples of individuals and groups of individuals who, we would now judge, were right to have flouted unjust laws, and who, in doing so, brought about social improvement. Legal judgements are made by the courts, but each of us, in the end, has to make our own ethical judgements. Ethics is in this sense an individual affair.

Medical ethics can also become politicized and function to serve particular political goals. We might talk about 'conservative medical ethics' or 'liberal medical ethics' in just this way. We believe that this politicized approach risks undermining the medical ethics enterprise. To take one kind of value as not open to being questioned because of one's political affiliation, or because of its dominant place in contemporary political discourse, is, to our minds, misguided. It risks foreclosing the terms of the debate, and preventing a proper consideration of all the reasons that ought to have force in the specific context.

The subject area of ethics has, for many centuries, been firmly placed in the discipline of philosophy. *Medical* ethics, being a division of ethics, might itself therefore reasonably be supposed also to be ultimately a branch of philosophy. This is indeed how many of the pioneers of medical ethics have seen it. Many doctors, and other healthcare professionals, have, however, resisted what might be called the supremacy of philosophy. Philosophers might take a particular medical case, or a medical situation, as a starting point, carry out philosophical analysis, and come to a conclusion about what, ethically, should be done. But healthcare professionals can feel frustrated by the answers: the philosophical analysis has failed to take into account the complexity of the *facts* of the case, and as a result the conclusion is too simplistic, and is *ethically* wrong. This interest in the details of the situation—in the empirical facts—has led to more systematic study of the empirical issues relevant to medical ethics over the last few decades—what some have called *the empirical turn* in medical ethics. Social scientists have got in on the act.

Research by medical sociologists and anthropologists has greatly enriched the subject of medical ethics. Often the research and analysis has given prominence to the lived experiences of patients, and especially of disempowered or marginalized people or groups, in order to tackle the injustices that these individuals face. Such research might show that an ethical analysis which concludes, for example, that in a specific situation the key ethical issue is that doctors should obtain 'informed consent' from patients, fails completely to tackle the most important ethically significant fact about the situation. For example, the research might show that the female patients in a particular context are not free to make their own decisions. Or that, for any of a number of reasons, patients do not have the power to do anything but follow the doctor's advice. Or that the central ethical issue is that most of those in need of medical help never get anywhere near a healthcare professional in the first place. The experiences both of people who could benefit from healthcare and of healthcare professionals, and the social, cultural, and political contexts of care, are often crucial to any ethical analysis aimed at informing practice. The social sciences are hugely important in ensuring that ethical analyses take properly into account all the facts that are relevant to actual practice. But, the facts alone can never simply 'speak for themselves'. Questions of what *ought* to be done in a specific situation or context are not answered by a knowledge

7

of the facts alone. Analysing what ought to be done and justifying the conclusion ultimately, in our view, involve philosophical analysis and coherent argument.

Some social scientists argue that any such analysis and any such argument are themselves grounded in a particular cultural and historical context, and that ethical principles themselves are relative to such context. On this view it could be problematic for a European, say, to pass judgement on the behaviour of the American doctor who participates in carrying out capital punishment, or the Somali doctor who undertakes female genital cutting on a young girl at the behest of her parents. Although this view does not render ethical argument redundant, it might undermine the idea that there is an ethical position that transcends any specific culture.

We resist this view. We believe that it can be appropriate to criticize healthcare practices that are widely accepted in a culture other than our own. We might, for example, be able to identify overarching values that give reason for judging that it would be wrong for a doctor to participate in capital punishment or female genital alteration: a value that transcends context and that could, rightly, motivate an intervention to change the behaviour of those who act in this way.

On the contributions of medical ethics

Medical ethics has many uses and our intention in this book is to showcase these uses across the nine chapters that follow. First, it can clarify conflicting views on what is the right thing to do. We might be uncertain about what a doctor needs to tell a patient before getting permission to carry out a specific medical procedure. Medical ethics will examine the kinds of information that will be appropriate to give to the patient; and come to a conclusion about what information ought to be disclosed in each specific situation.

Second, medical ethics, like Socrates, can operate as a gadfly: standing back, analysing the situation, and provoking those in the situation to act differently. In these instances, medical ethics has critiqued conventional practice and thinking, and found it wanting.

Third, medical ethics can identify gaps in current knowledge and can highlight the kinds of research needed to support good medical practice. Ethical analysis might, for example, identify gaps, crucial to making an ethically right decision, in our understanding of what is happening in a medical situation, drawing attention to the need for further empirical evidence to settle the question about how a doctor should act in that particular instance.

Fourth, medical ethics can act as a crutch: a form of practical support to those who have to make difficult decisions—the healthcare professionals, and sometimes patients themselves and their families. However experienced the doctor, or other healthcare professional, ethical problems do arise that are highly problematic and that may raise difficult emotions. The discipline of medical ethics can act as support and guide in clarifying the steps to be taken in coming to a decision. This discipline involves: seeing how an ethical issue arises in practice, carefully collecting evidence about the relevant facts and values that concern that issue for all those involved, using those facts and values to clarify the arguments, and, by a process of reasoning through the various options, coming to a decision as to how to act.

In this book, we discuss these contributions across different areas: genetics, modern reproductive technologies, resource allocation, mental health, medical research, and so on. At the end of the book we guide the reader to other issues and further reading on each of these areas. Across the chapters, we will illustrate the different ways in which medical ethics can be put to use. The one perspective that is common to all the chapters is the central importance of reasoning and argument. We believe that medical ethics is essentially a rational subject: that is, it is all about giving reasons for the views that you take, and being prepared to change your views on the basis of reasons and evidence. That is why Chapter 3 is a reflection on various tools of rational argument: reasoning is not owned solely by well-trained philosophers. We can all improve our reasoning skills and adopt tools to assist us in developing the quality of our ethical arguments.

Although we believe in the central importance of reasons and evidence, even here the voice of the fox in us sounds a note of caution. Clear thinking and high standards of rationality are not enough. We need to develop our hearts as well as our minds. Consistency and moral enthusiasm can lead to bad acts and wrong decisions if pursued without the right sensitivities, and the right awareness of the context in which decisions are enacted. The novelist, Zadie Smith, has written: 'There is no bigger crime, in the English comic novel, than thinking you are right. The lesson of the comic novel is that our moral enthusiasms make us inflexible, one-dimensional, flat.' This is a lesson we need to take into any area of practice where values are disputed, including medical ethics.

What better place to begin our tour of medical ethics than at the end, with the thorny issue of euthanasia?

Chapter 2
Assisted dying: good medical practice, or murder?

The practice of euthanasia—killing a patient for the patient's benefit—contradicts one of the oldest and most venerated of moral injunctions: 'Thou shalt not kill'. The practice of euthanasia, under some circumstances, is morally required by the two most widely regarded principles for guiding good medical practice: respect for patient autonomy and promoting patients' best interests.

Euthanasia is one form of what is generally termed *assisted dying*. Other forms include assisting suicide and the withholding or withdrawing of life-extending medical treatment. The laws on euthanasia vary across countries. In the Netherlands and Belgium euthanasia may, under certain conditions, be carried out within the law. In Switzerland, and in a small number of US states, physician-assisted suicide, that cousin of euthanasia, is legal, again if certain conditions are met. Four times in the last hundred years the UK Parliament has given careful consideration to legalizing either mercy killing or assisting suicide, and on each occasion has rejected the possibility. Throughout the world, societies founded to promote voluntary euthanasia attract large numbers of members.

In this chapter we will argue the case in favour of the law allowing health professionals, under certain conditions, to assist patients to die. In so doing we will illustrate one common and powerful method of argument: *countering the counter-arguments*.

We begin by laying the groundwork for our approach by using four of what we call *tools* of ethical reasoning. Further tools will be discussed in Chapter 3.

Logic

There is a common, but invalid, argument against assisted dying: 'playing the Nazi card'. This card is played when the opponent of assisted dying says to the supporter of assisted dying: 'Your views are just like those of the Nazis'. There is no need for the opponent to spell out the rhetorical conclusion: 'and therefore your views are totally immoral'.

In assessing an argument it can be useful to summarize it in logical form (see Figure 2): in terms of premises, and the conclusion that is supposed to follow, logically, from those premises. This

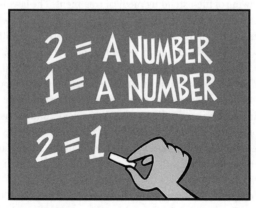

2. **Beware false logic.**

form is known as a *syllogism*. When presented as a syllogism, the Nazi card argument looks like this:

Premise 1:   Many views held by Nazis are totally immoral.

Premise 2:   Your view (support for assisted dying under some circumstances) is one view held by Nazis.

Conclusion: Your view is totally immoral.

This is not a valid argument. It would be valid only if *all* the views held by Nazis were immoral.

We will therefore replace premise 1 by premise 1* as follows:

Premise 1*:   All views held by Nazis are totally immoral.

In this case the argument is *logically valid*, but in order to assess whether the argument is *true* we need to assess the truth of premise 1*.

There are two possible interpretations of premise 1*. One interpretation is a version of the classic *false* argument known as *argumentum ad hominem* (or *bad company fallacy*). Warburton describes this fallacy as stating that a particular view is true or false, not because of the reasons in favour or against the view, but by virtue of the fact that a particular person (or group of people) holds that view. But bad people may hold some good views, and good people may hold some bad views. It is quite possible that a senior Nazi was vegetarian on moral grounds. This fact (if it is a fact) is irrelevant to the question of whether there are, or are not, moral grounds in favour of vegetarianism. What is important are the reasons for and against the particular view, not the person who holds it. Hitler's well-known vegetarianism, by the way, was on health, not on moral, grounds (see Spencer, 1996).

The other, more promising, interpretation of premise 1* is that those views that are categorized as 'Nazi views' are all immoral. The Nazi views being referred to are a set of related views, all immoral, that are driven by racism and involve killing people against both their will and their interests. Thus, when it is said that assisted dying is a Nazi view, what is meant is that it is one of these core immoral views that characterize the immoral Nazi worldview. The problem with this argument, however, is that most supporters of assisted dying—as it is practised in the Netherlands for example—are not supporting the Nazi worldview. Quite the contrary. Those on both sides of the assisted dying debate agree that the Nazi killings that took place under the guise of 'euthanasia' were grossly immoral. The point at issue in the debate is whether assisted dying in certain specific circumstances is right or wrong, moral or immoral. All depends on being clear about these specific circumstances and being precise about what is meant by euthanasia. Only then can the arguments for and against legalizing assisted dying be properly evaluated. What is needed, for a start, are definitions of key terms.

Defining terms

Let us begin with some definitions relevant to debates over assisted dying in the medical setting (Box 1). The purpose of these definitions is twofold: to make distinctions between different kinds of assisted dying, distinctions that may be ethically significant; and to provide us with a precise vocabulary. If a word is used in one sense at one point in the argument, and in another sense at another point, then the argument may look valid when in fact it is not.

If you study Box 1 it will be immediately clear that playing the Nazi card rides roughshod over some important distinctions. The various types of assisted dying relevant to medical practice all require that the doctor's action is for the patient's benefit or that the patient competently refuses treatment. Furthermore, there are many types of assisted dying, and in assessing the arguments, it will be important to see how they apply to each type. What the Nazis practised was *involuntary* killing—*not*

Box 1 Assisted dying: some terms and definitions

Euthanasia (what used to be called *active euthanasia* and is often called *mercy killing*)

X performs an action that intentionally kills Y, for Y's benefit.

Voluntary euthanasia

Euthanasia when Y competently requests the action which results in Y's death with the intention that it will lead to Y's death.

Non-voluntary euthanasia

Euthanasia when Y is not competent to express a preference regarding the action which results in Y's death, e.g. Y is a severely disabled newborn child.

Involuntary euthanasia

X performs euthanasia, despite the fact that this is contrary to Y's expressed wishes.

Withholding treatment (what used to be called *passive euthanasia*)

X allows Y to die by withholding life-prolonging treatment. This might be because X believes that withholding treatment is for Y's benefit, or because Y competently refuses the treatment.

Withdrawing treatment (what used to be called *passive euthanasia* even though it involves actively withdrawing treatment)

X allows Y to die by withdrawing life-prolonging treatment. This might be because X believes that withdrawing treatment is for Y's benefit, or because Y competently refuses continuation of the treatment.

(continued)

Box 1 Continued

Suicide

Y intentionally kills himself.

Assisted suicide

X intentionally helps Y to kill himself.

Physician-assisted suicide

X (a physician) intentionally helps Y to kill himself.

euthanasia, as the killings were not to each person's benefit: it was none of the types of assisted dying that are relevant to medical practice.

Medical ethics is not, however, a purely theoretical discipline. It serves a *practical* purpose. It is about what we ought to do in a particular set of circumstances. Clarifying the facts of the matter as they arise in a particular setting is as important as clarifying terms: what action is being proposed; why is it being proposed; and what effects will that action have?

Elucidating concepts

The application of some concepts in medical ethics to some situations may require more than a definition. A good example is that of the *best interests* of a patient—a concept used extensively in law and in everyday medical care and closely related to the idea of patient benefit which is used in the definition of euthanasia (see Box 1).

In the context of assisted dying an important question is: can it be in the best interests of a patient to die? We believe it can.

The courts believe it can. Most doctors, nurses, and relatives believe it can. The question arises quite frequently in healthcare. A patient with an incurable and fatal disease may reach a stage where she will die within a day or two, but could be kept alive, with active treatment, for a few weeks more. This situation might occur, for example, because the patient gets a chest infection in addition to the underlying fatal disease. Antibiotics might treat this acute problem although they will do nothing to stop the progress of the underlying disease. All those caring for the patient will often agree that it is in the patient's best interests to die now rather than receive life-extending treatment. This is particularly likely if the patient's quality of life is very poor, perhaps because of sustained and untreatable difficulty in breathing. Assessing best interests requires close attention to be paid to specific facts about the patient's current experiences.

Not everyone agrees, however, that it can be in someone's best interests to die. Some would argue that we never know what a patient's quality of life is like, especially if the patient is unable to communicate effectively, for example due to a stroke. It might be further argued that we can never predict how the patient's quality of life will be affected by treatment. A problem with such scepticism, however, is that it does not help us to decide what to do: whether to prolong the life with treatment or not. It leaves us paralysed with indecision.

A further issue is uncertainty over the nature of the experience of being dead. Those who believe that there is some kind of afterlife would need to compare the experience of the patient if kept alive with the presumed likely experience after death. For those who believe that there is no experience after death then the question of whether it is in a person's best interests to die would reduce to the question of whether her likely experience, were she to be kept alive, would overall be so bad that no experience at all would be better. The experiences of severe pain or distress, continuing until death, might be examples of life worse than death.

Some claim that it is always in a person's best interests to be alive rather than dead. It is difficult, however, to justify such a view in the light of some examples of suffering.

Even if we believe that it would be in a person's best interests to die, even if the person wishes to die, and even if we believe that it would be right to withhold, and perhaps withdraw, life-extending treatment, we may still believe that it would be wrong to actively *kill* the person. Let's explore this through *case comparison*.

Case comparison

Case comparison involves comparing two (or more) cases that are similar in many ways. If, for example, you are uncertain what is the right thing to do in a particular situation, you could consider a somewhat similar case but one in which you are more certain about what is right. In comparing the cases you might ask yourself two questions: are there any *morally relevant* differences between the cases? And, do these morally relevant differences justify treating the cases differently? The fundamental logical point is of *consistency*: we are being inconsistent if we treat two cases differently, unless there is a (morally) relevant difference between them.

In the debates over assisted dying an interesting pair of cases to compare are medical situations involving withholding (and perhaps withdrawing) life-sustaining treatment with those involving (active) voluntary euthanasia—with killing the patient. Thus we might compare Case 1 and Case 2 in Box 2 and Box 3.

In Case 1, the doctor's withholding treatment is widely accepted as morally right and is protected by law in many countries, including England.

Box 2 Case 1: prostate cancer

A 92-year-old man with prostate cancer, whose life could be extended by several months (but no more) by an operation and chemotherapy, refuses these treatments and asks only to be kept comfortable and out of pain. His doctor respects his refusal of treatment. The patient dies within a few days.

Box 3 Case 2: the Dr Cox case

Lillian Boyes was a 70-year-old patient with very severe rheumatoid arthritis. The pain seemed to be beyond the reach of pain-killers. She was expected to die within a matter of days or weeks. She asked her doctor, Dr Cox, to kill her. Dr Cox injected her with a lethal dose of potassium chloride.

In Case 2, which is a real case that reached the English courts, Dr Cox was found guilty of the serious criminal offence of attempted murder. The judge, in directing the jury, said:

> Even the prosecution case acknowledged that he [Dr Cox]…was prompted by deep distress at Lillian Boyes' condition; by a belief that she was totally beyond recall and by an intense compassion for her fearful suffering. Nonetheless…if he injected her with potassium chloride for the primary purpose of killing her, or hastening her death, he is guilty of the offence charged…neither the express wishes of the patient nor of her loving and devoted family can affect the position.

Dr Cox was found guilty.

This case clearly established that (active) euthanasia is illegal (and potentially murder) under English common law even when voluntary. The reason, by the way, why Dr Cox was charged with *attempted* murder (and not murder) was that the prosecution believed that an English jury would not convict him of murder (which would carry a mandatory life sentence).

The key difference between Cases 1 and 2, on which much legal and moral weight is placed, is that Dr Cox *killed* Lilian Boyes, and did not simply allow her to die.

Making an argument by countering the counter-arguments

Medical ethics is about *reasoned argument* just as the technical aspects of medicine are about *assessing scientific evidence*. How does one construct a reasoned argument? One powerful way has three steps:

Step 1:   Propose what you think is the morally best decision or course of action—and specify the main reason(s) or arguments why you think so.

Step 2:   Articulate as many counter-arguments to that proposed decision as you can.

Step 3:   Consider each counter-argument in turn and think whether there is a counter to that counter-argument.

If all the counter-arguments are effectively countered then you have constructed a reasoned argument in favour of your original position. If you cannot counter all of the identified counter-arguments then you will need to re-think your original decision or course of action.

It is noteworthy that no argument is truly 'watertight'. No argument is the last word. It is always possible that you have missed a possible counter-argument to your original proposed decision, or that there is a counter to your counter to a counter-argument. Ethics, no less than science, is, at root, an exercise of the imagination requiring not only precision but also creative intelligence.

We will illustrate the process of reasoned argument by consideration of the case of Dr Cox in Case 2.

Step 1: propose a decision and the main reason(s) in its favour

We propose that Dr Cox made the morally right decision in killing Lilian Boyes. The two principal reasons in favour of this view are:

1. That it was in Lilian Boyes' best interests to be killed: the suffering that she would otherwise have experienced for the remainder of her life made living worse than death.
2. That Lilian Boyes' own decision was that she wished to be killed, and she was fully competent to make that decision.

Step 2: articulate counter-examples to the proposed decision

We will consider eight counter-arguments.

1. In trying to kill Lilian Boyes, Dr Cox may cause her more suffering than if he had not attempted to kill her.
2. There may be a slim chance that Lilian Boyes, if she is not killed, will recover sufficiently from the arthritis to live with little or no suffering. Killing her prevents that possibility.
3. It is not fair on Dr Cox: he will bear the guilt of having killed Lilian Boyes.
4. Even if, in this case, it seems right to have killed Lilian Boyes, it would still have been wrong to do so; for unless we keep strictly to the rule that killing is wrong, we will slide down a slippery slope. Soon doctors will be killing patients when they

mistakenly believe it is in patients' best interests. And doctors may slip further and kill patients in the interests of themselves or of patients' relatives.

5. Dr Cox, whatever his own personal moral beliefs, should not have killed Lilian Boyes because to do so was illegal.

6. The argument from Nature: that whereas withholding or withdrawing treatment from a dying patient is allowing nature to take its course; killing is an interference in nature, and therefore wrong.

7. The argument from Playing God: killing is taking on a role that should be reserved for God alone. Letting die, on the other hand, is not usurping God's role, and may, when done with care and love, be enabling God's will to be fulfilled.

8. Killing is in principle a (great) wrong. The difference between withholding or withdrawing treatment, on the one hand, and (active) euthanasia, on the other hand, is fundamentally that the former involves 'allowing to die' and the latter involves killing; and killing is wrong—it is a fundamental wrong.

Step 3: counter (if you can) the counter-arguments

Let us consider each of these eight counter-arguments in turn.

1. This argument is not an argument that euthanasia—mercy killing—is wrong in principle, but that in the real world we can never be sure it will be merciful. There are three possible situations:

   a. Dr Cox does not inject potassium chloride into Lilian Boyes. She dies 'naturally' having suffered a considerable amount of pain—let us call this amount 'X'.

   b. Dr Cox kills Lilian Boyes with the intended outcome. She dies almost instantaneously and almost painlessly. In this case Lilian Boyes will suffer an amount Y where Y is much smaller than X, perhaps zero.

c.   Dr Cox tries to kill Lilian Boyes with potassium chloride but fails and the injection leads to greater suffering for Lilian Boyes: an amount of suffering Z, where Z is greater than X.

It is because of possibility (c), according to argument 1, that it would be better that Dr Cox does not try to kill Lilian Boyes.

We can now compare the situation where Dr Cox simply allows Lilian Boyes to die with the situation where he gives her the injection of potassium chloride. In the former case the total amount of suffering is X. In the latter case the amount of suffering is either Y (close to zero) or Z (greater than X). If what is important is avoiding suffering, then whether it is better for Dr Cox to give the injection or not depends on the differences between X, Y, and Z and the probabilities of each of these outcomes occurring. If almost instantaneous death (scenario (b)) is by far the most likely result from giving the injection, and if the suffering level X is significantly more than Y, then it would seem right to give the injection because the chances are very much in favour of this leading to significantly less suffering.

If uncertainty over outcomes were a reason not to act we would either be completely paralysed in making decisions or frequently, through our inaction, fail to do good. We conclude that argument 1 does not provide a convincing argument against what Dr Cox did, nor, more generally, against the legalization of euthanasia.

2.   Argument 2 suffers the same weakness as argument 1. In order to judge Lilian Boyes' best interests we need to consider the various possible outcomes, the quality of life that each of these would entail, and the probabilities of each occurring. How much weight we give to the possibility that Lilian Boyes will make a spectacular recovery from her arthritis, and the consequent pain and discomfort, depends crucially on

the probability of this happening. If it is very unlikely, as indeed it was, then argument 2 is not persuasive.

A possible counter to this counter-argument is that although Lilian Boyes' almost miraculous recovery is very unlikely the weight to be given to this remote possibility should be infinite. There are three responses to this argument: first, what grounds are there for giving *infinite* weight to the possibility of recovery? Second, there is also a remote possibility that giving the potassium chloride, although intended to kill Lilian Boyes, might in fact miraculously cure her (some medical discoveries occur when an intervention has a very different result from what is expected). Third, if argument 2 provides a convincing reason for rejecting (active) euthanasia, it also provides a convincing reason for rejecting the withholding of medical treatment in all circumstances.

Arguments 1 and 2 fail, ultimately, because the chances of recovery are not being assessed in the same evidence-based way as the chances that the patient will not recover. Possible harms and benefits must be assessed on an equal footing: getting the facts right is crucial to making good ethical judgements.

3. The third argument fails because it begs the very question that is under debate. Dr Cox should feel guilt only if killing Lilian Boyes were the wrong thing to do. We first have to answer the question of what is the right thing to do and only then can we ask whether we ought to feel guilt. Some people may *feel* guilt even when they believe that their action was morally right. Over time, such feelings are likely to be minimized by the belief in the rightness of the action. In any case, it is up to Dr Cox to decide whether or not he is willing, in pursuance of what he believes is the morally right action, to bear the burden of guilt (if indeed he feels any).

4. Argument 4 is a version of what is known as the 'slippery slope argument'. This is such an important type of argument

in medical ethics that we will consider it in detail, and how it applies to Dr Cox's actions, in Chapter 3.

5. The fact that an action is illegal does normally count as a (moral) reason not to do it, which is in some way to be weighed against other moral considerations. Argument 5 might therefore be a strong argument for why Dr Cox should not have acted as he did. It is, however, no argument at all against the more interesting question of whether what he did should or should not be illegal in the first place.

6 and 7. The arguments from Nature and from Playing God have, like the slippery slope argument, a more general application in medical ethics. We will consider them in Chapter 3, and show why we do not think that these counter-arguments are convincing.

8. Of all the arguments considered, it is only argument 8 that views killing as wrong in principle.

But how can we examine the morality of a basic principle such as *killing is (always) wrong*? One way is through further case comparisons, for example to consider whether killing in war is always wrong. If it isn't then the principle that killing is *always* wrong needs to be revised. What looked like a basic principle may become more complex, more nuanced, and in need of further justification. If killing is not always wrong, why is it wrong in the case of euthanasia?

Opponents of the legalization of euthanasia may ultimately rest their case on the one basic principle that *killing is morally wrong*. They may accept that there are difficult cases (e.g. in war) when killing one person may save another—or many others. But in the case of mercy killing, no other person's life will be saved.

If we are to convince opponents of the legalization of euthanasia that they are wrong, then in addition to countering the counter-arguments we will need to give some account of why their basic principle that killing is wrong is generally valid, but not in this case. We might argue, for example, that it is right that we have a strong intuition that killing is wrong. For most people dying now would be a great harm compared with continuing to live. The reason why killing is normally a great wrong is that dying is normally a great harm. The wrong of killing, however, is a result of the harm of dying, not vice versa. If, therefore, it is in the best interests of a patient to die now rather than suffer a prolonged and painful dying, and if, further, the patient wishes to be killed, then killing is no longer a wrong. When death is a benefit, and not a harm, and is desired by the person, then killing is not a wrong. Those who argue that mercy killing is wrong in principle, forget the conceptual link between the wrong of killing and the harm of dying.

Countering the counter-arguments is often, as here, quite a long process as it attempts to be meticulous. It is therefore helpful to conclude your case with a brief account of where, at root, you think your opponents are going wrong. We will illustrate this by concluding our case in favour of the legalization of euthanasia. As you will see we end with a rhetorical flourish. Do you think that the final sentence of this chapter makes a fair point or do you think that it is unscrupulous rhetoric?

Our conclusion is that we reject the view that voluntary euthanasia is wrong in principle on the grounds that this argument puts the cart before the horse: it is the harm of dying that makes killing a wrong and not the other way round. When suffering is the result of following a moral principle then we need to look very carefully at our moral principle and ask whether we are applying it too inflexibly. We believe this is what those who claim that voluntary euthanasia is morally wrong are doing. It is perverse to seek a sense of moral purity when this is gained at the expense of the suffering of others.

Chapter 3
A toolbox of reasoning

Doctors, nurses, and other health professionals will normally have good reasons for doing what they do. It would be foolish not to give careful consideration to what experienced practitioners do and think is right. But the role of philosophy, and its application in medical ethics, is to demand reasons and to subject these reasons to careful analysis. Medical practice should be continually improving through subjecting itself to the scrutiny of those twin disciplines, science and philosophy. Science asks: what is the evidence that this is the indicated course of care and treatment? Philosophy asks: what are the reasons for the moral choices made?

In Chapter 2 we highlighted four tools of ethical reasoning. In this chapter we will discuss a further four in some detail (see Box 4) and will end with a glimpse of what lies beyond them.

Box 4 Eight tools of ethical reasoning

1. Distinguishing facts from values
2. Reasoning from principles
3. Defining terms (see Chapter 2)
4. Elucidating concepts (see Chapter 2 and the discussion of *best interests* in this chapter)

(continued)

Box 4 Continued

5. Case comparison (see Chapter 2)
6. Thought experiments
7. Logic (see Chapter 2)
8. Spotting and avoiding fallacies in reasoning

Box 5 Case 1: home or hospital care?

Mr P is an 80-year-old man with severe Alzheimer's disease and long-standing lung disease. He is cared for at home by his 82-year-old wife. He requires oxygen at home and has frequent chest infections for which he receives antibiotics. With his most recent chest infection, he has not responded well to antibiotic tablets and his general condition is deteriorating. It is possible that with hospital treatment, including intravenous antibiotics and physiotherapy, he may recover from this infection although he is bound to develop a similar infection again in the near future. Admission to hospital in the past has caused him distress because he does not cope well with changing environments. His wife, however, says that she thinks that he should go to hospital so he can be given maximum treatment. Should Mr P's doctor admit him to hospital?

Let's begin, as medical ethicists so often do, with a clinical case before systematically laying out our eight tools of ethical reasoning. This is presented in Box 5.

Tool 1: distinguishing facts from values

The first tool of ethical reasoning is identifying and distinguishing the facts and the values at stake in the situation. The distinction is important because the evaluation of *facts* generally requires an *assessment of evidence* about the way the world is, for example which particular medication provides the highest probability of cure for a particular disease; or how does this disease affect people's experiences. The evaluation of ethical *values* generally requires *ethical argument*. Consider buying a new car. Suppose, for Person A, safety and reliability are key—they are A's *values*. Suppose, for Person B, performance and comfort are most important. For A, the relevant *facts* about different types of car are their safety and reliability. For B, it is evidence about performance and comfort that is important. One point that we wish to emphasize and that is illustrated by this example is that it is our values that determine which facts are relevant and not vice versa: values are primary.

So how does this distinction between facts and values apply to Case 1 in Box 5? The values at stake include maximizing Mr P's *best interests*, respecting his likely *previous wishes*, perhaps respecting his *current wishes*, and being *fair* to Mr P's wife. The relevant facts follow from these values. What is his current quality of life (relevant to his *best interests*)? What is the probability that the antibiotics will improve his quality of life? What is the impact on his quality of life of the distress caused by hospital admission? How capable is he of understanding the key issues and making his own decision? If he is no longer capable, what might his views have been about this situation had he discussed them before he lost such capability? What is the burden of care on Mr P's wife, and what are her views?

Facts and values are frequently confused in ethical discussions. Consider an issue of medical confidentiality. A patient consults her doctor following two episodes of fits. The doctor initiates investigations to determine the cause and informs the patient that the law requires her to stop driving and to inform the driving authorities of the fits. Two weeks later the doctor sees the patient driving. Should the doctor inform the authorities? In England there is no legal duty for the doctor to do so.

Suppose that Person C thinks that the doctor should breach confidentiality, and Person D thinks the doctor should not breach confidentiality. Do C and D differ with regard to their ethical *values*? Not necessarily. Both may believe that the overriding value is to minimize road deaths overall. C thinks this will be achieved by doctors informing on patients. D believes that overall if doctors inform it will discourage patients who have had a fit from seeking medical help, resulting in more drivers with uncontrolled epilepsy and more road deaths. C and D agree about the appropriate ethical value but disagree about the facts. Suppose Person E believes that the doctor should not inform the authorities because for E the overriding ethical value is that doctors should respect the autonomy and confidentiality of patients. D and E agree about what the doctor should do, but disagree over the relevant ethical values.

Tool 2: reasoning from principles

Several books and many articles organize the analysis of medical ethics around four principles and their scope of application (see Box 6). These principles might best be seen as perspectives that capture four broad ethical values that underpin good medical practice rather than as the premises of a logical argument.

Box 6 Four principles in medical ethics

1. Respect for patient autonomy

According to Gillon, autonomy (literally self-rule) is the capacity to think, decide, and act on the basis of such thought and decision, freely and independently. Respect for patient autonomy requires health professionals (and others, including the patient's family) to help patients to come to their own decisions (e.g. by providing important information) and to respect and follow those decisions (even when the health professional believes that the patient's decision is wrong).

2. Beneficence: the promotion of what is best for the patient

This principle emphasizes the moral importance of doing good to others and, particularly in the medical context, doing good to patients. Following this principle would entail doing what was best for the patient. This raises the question of who should be the judge of what is best for the patient. This principle is often interpreted as focusing on what an objective assessment by a relevant health professional would determine as being in the patient's best interests. The patient's own views are captured by the principle of respect for patient autonomy.

The two principles conflict when a competent patient chooses a course of action which is not in her best interests.

3. Non-maleficence: avoiding harm

This principle is the other side of the coin of the principle of beneficence. It states that we should not harm patients. In most situations this principle does not add anything useful to the principle of beneficence. The main reason for retaining the principle of non-maleficence is that it is generally thought that we have a prima facie duty not to harm anyone, whereas we owe a duty of beneficence to a limited number of people only.

4. Justice

There are four components to this principle: distributive justice; respect for the law; rights; and retributive justice.

With regard to distributive justice this principle emphasizes two points: first, that patients in similar situations should normally have access to the same healthcare; and, second, that in determining what level of healthcare should be available for one set of patients we must take into account the effect of such a use of resources on other patients. In other words, we must try to distribute our limited resources (time, money, intensive care beds) fairly.

In thinking about Case 1 in Box 5 we will first consider the principle of respect for patient autonomy. From this perspective a key question is whether Mr P himself can make the decision? Has he sufficient ability to understand and weigh the issues relevant to home or hospital care? If he hasn't, do we have any past evidence about whether he would have wanted home or hospital care?

If Mr P cannot make the decision, we can turn to the principle of beneficence. This emphasizes that we should act in Mr P's best interests. We talked a bit about best interests in Chapter 2. If acting in a person's best interests is promoting his well-being we can draw on the three common approaches to what is meant by *well-being*. The first, known as *mental-state theory*, is that our well-being is determined by our mental experiences: that the experiences of pleasure and happiness are the positive aspects of well-being; and that misery and pain are negative aspects. Our well-being is given by the amount of positive experiences minus the negative experiences. A second approach is called *desire-fulfilment theory*: well-being consists in having our desires fulfilled. On this view best interests and respecting autonomy are very similar. A third approach, called *objective list theory*, sees well-being as multi-dimensional and where the dimensions are not determined by each individual but are intrinsic to the idea of well-being. On this view, we need to come to some agreement about what comprises the objectively good features of human existence. Certain things, deep personal relationships or the development of one's abilities for example, are commonly seen as contributing to well-being, whether or not they are desired and whether or not they lead to pleasurable mental states. Conversely certain things, such as being deceived or gaining pleasure from cruelty, for example, are seen to reduce well-being even if they lead to pleasurable mental states, or are desired.

It is not entirely clear what it is that is in Mr P's best interests. However, applying the principle of beneficence identifies some of the important issues on which we should make a judgement: how much distress and suffering is hospital admission likely to cause him; how positive or negative are his current experiences, and his likely experiences after hospital treatment; and what he would have desired in this situation? Objective list theory might highlight the negative aspects of the damage caused by Alzheimer's disease. Even if he enjoys life from day to day one might argue that his well-being is severely compromised by the brain damage and consequent impaired ability to understand and think. Assessing his well-being, on this view, may crucially depend on facts about how the Alzheimer's disease has affected his cognitive abilities.

What weight should doctors put on the views of Mr P's wife? From the perspective of the principle of beneficence her views are relevant because she is in a good position to understand what is in Mr P's best interests. From the perspective of respect for patient autonomy her views are relevant either because she might know what Mr P would have wanted, or because Mr P might (when competent) have wanted his wife to make decisions about his care. Neither principle, however, gives Mr P's wife the right to make the decision simply because she is his wife.

The principle of justice highlights further issues. Unless the hospital care is paid for entirely by Mr P then the question arises as to whether providing such care is fair to others given competing demands on hospital resources. Conversely, if Mr P remains at home, does an unfair (and unwanted) burden of care fall on his wife?

Tools 3 and 4: defining terms; and elucidating concepts

It is always important in ethical discussion to be clear what we mean by the words we use. Sometimes a simple definition will suffice (e.g. *euthanasia* in Chapter 2, Box 1), but often we need to analyse what is meant by a word in more detail (as we have just done for the term *well-being*). Even though the difference is one of degree, not of kind, it is worth distinguishing tools 3 and 4, as we did in Chapter 2. This is because in ethical argument it can be useful to ask the two questions: are both sides in the argument working with the same *definitions* of key terms? And, what does each side understand by the words used in the definitions? For example, in debates about assisted dying it will be important that both sides agree the definition of *euthanasia*, and it will also be important to establish what each side means by the concept of patient *benefit* (which is used in the definition).

Tool 5: case comparison

In Chapter 2, we discussed the value of comparing *real* cases in ethical argument. Philosophers frequently use imaginary, even unrealistic, situations known as *thought experiments*. We will consider the use of thought experiments as a separate tool.

Tool 6: thought experiments

Imaginary cases can be used as part of a case comparison, or they can be used to test our principles and arguments. One of the uses of the imagination in ethical reasoning is in thinking of thought experiments that take the argument forward, or that challenge our routine ways of thinking.

One famous thought experiment (the *experience machine*) was put forward by Robert Nozick. His purpose was to criticize the mental state theory of well-being (see 'Tool 2: reasoning from principles'). This thought experiment uses ideas from science fiction. This is presented in Box 7.

Nozick argues that we should not plug in because there are aspects of life that are important to us over and above mental states. For example, he suggests, we want to *do* certain things (write this book for example) and not simply have the experience of (apparently) writing the book; and that we want to *be* a certain type of person, which involves doing and interacting with others and the world in a way that we don't do if we are plugged into the machine. Nozick's experience machine thought experiment has become a main tool for those ethicists who seek to argue against mental state theories of well-being.

Tool 7: logic

In Chapter 2, when presenting the Nazi card argument as a syllogism, we noted that an argument can be logically invalid. Such *logically* invalid arguments are one type of fallacious reasoning. Many other fallacies in reasoning are less formal. These are fallacies either because the premises are unsound or because the connections between the premises are inadequate to make a sound argument. Our final tool in ethical reasoning concerns such fallacies.

Tool 8: spotting and avoiding fallacies in reasoning

Logicians like to spot, and name, fallacious arguments rather as ornithologists spot birds. We came across the *argumentum ad hominem* in Chapter 2. Spotting fallacies, and learning how to avoid them, is a useful exercise in medical ethics because it helps us to see through a rhetorically powerful, but ultimately false, argument. We will discuss five such fallacies. For further fallacies, see Warburton.

The no-true Scotsman move (after Flew, 1989)

> Someone says: 'No Scotsman would beat his wife to a shapeless pulp with a blunt instrument'. He is confronted with a falsifying instance: 'Mr Angus McSporran did just that'. Instead of withdrawing, or at least qualifying, the too rash original claim our patriot insists: 'Well, no *true* Scotsman would do such a thing!'

What seems to be a statement of fact (an empirical claim) is made impervious to counter-examples by adapting the meaning of the words so that the statement becomes true by definition and empty of any empirical content.

The ten-leaky-buckets tactic (after Flew, 1989)

This tactic involves 'presenting a series of several unsound arguments as if their mere conjunction might render them collectively valid'. The analogy here is that if you want to carry water successfully over a distance, leaky buckets will not do no matter how many you have, as you will lose a lot of the water. What you need is one, or more, intact buckets.

It is common for people to defend a view on a particular subject with several poor arguments and to somehow think that because they have given several arguments they have provided a powerful justification for their view. What is needed, however, is one (or more) *sound* argument. The fact that the critic of euthanasia can produce several arguments in favour of that view does not amount to a defence of the position if all those arguments are invalid (see Chapter 2).

Many invalid *arguments*, no matter how many, cannot add up to a valid argument. This situation needs to be distinguished, however, from the accumulation of *evidence*, where every item possesses some weight in its own right.

The argument from nature

We briefly met this fallacy, and the following one, in Chapter 2. The argument from nature boils down to the assertion: this is not natural therefore it is morally wrong. The argument has been used against homosexuality, and it is often brought out in the contexts of assisted dying, modern reproductive technologies, and genetics. The argument is problematic in at least three ways. First, it is not clear what it means to say that something is unnatural. If 10 per cent of humans are predominantly homosexual, and homosexual behaviour is seen in other species, what is meant by saying that homosexuality is unnatural? Second, it seems quite unclear why it should follow from the fact that something is unnatural, that it is morally wrong. What kind of reason could be given in support of this? Third, there are an enormous number of counter-examples, not least from medical practice itself, to the claim that what is unnatural is morally wrong. The life of a child with meningitis may be saved by antibiotics and intensive care. Neither treatment is 'natural' on any meaning that can be given to that term, but we don't consider either to be morally wrong.

The argument from playing God

This argument involves first identifying an act as one that amounts to 'playing God' and second making the assertion that it is morally wrong because only God has the right to perform it. The argument is problematic in ways analogous to the 'argument from nature'. What criteria can be used to distinguish between our carrying out God's will, and our usurping his role? Which of the following is playing God: providing IVF; withdrawing life support; injecting antibiotics; transplanting a kidney? First, we have to decide which acts are right or wrong before we can determine those that might be described as playing God. The concept of playing God is therefore of no help in determining what it is right to do; it is merely a rhetorical attempt to strengthen an argument without good reason.

The slippery slope arguments

The core of slippery slope arguments is that once you accept one particular position then it will be extremely difficult, or indeed impossible, not to accept more and more extreme positions that are morally wrong—extremely difficult, that is, not to slip down the slope all the way to the bottom. If you do not want to accept the more extreme positions you must not accept the original, less extreme position.

There are two types of slippery slope argument: the logical type and the empirical type. The logical type is simply fallacious. The empirical type makes an empirical claim—a factual claim about how the world is—and therefore requires empirical (scientific) evidence, and not simply ethical argument, if it is to be justified.

The logical type of slippery slope argument consists in three steps:

Step 1:   The claim that as a matter of logic, if you accept the (apparently reasonable) proposition p, then you must also accept the closely related proposition q. Similarly, if you accept q you must accept proposition r; and so on through propositions s, t, etc. Propositions p, q, r, s, t, etc. form a series of related propositions such that adjacent propositions are more similar to each other than those further apart in the series.

Step 2:   This involves showing, or gaining agreement from the other side, that at some stage in this series the propositions become morally unacceptable, or false.

Step 3:   This involves applying formal logic as follows. If the first proposition (p) were morally acceptable then the later proposition (t) would also be morally acceptable. But since we are agreed that the later proposition (t) is *not* morally acceptable, we must conclude that the first proposition (p) is also *not* morally acceptable.

In summary, Step 1 is to establish the premise: *if p then t*. Step 2 is to establish the premise: *t is false*. Step 3 is to point out that from these premises it follows, logically, that *p is false*.

This logical form of slippery slope argument is related closely to a class of paradoxes known as the 'sorites paradoxes' first identified by the ancient Greeks. The name 'sorites' comes from the Greek 'soros' meaning a heap. An early example of this type of paradox involved arguing that one grain of sand does not make a heap, and adding one grain of sand to something that is not a heap will not make a heap, so you can never have a heap of sand. A casual observation of children playing on the beach will show that the logical form of slippery slope argument is fallacious. The fallacy lies in Step 1. Although propositions p and q may be so close that any moral difference is small, and perhaps imperceptible, there is still that small difference. And although we can break the large distance between proposition p and t into a large number of very small and (almost) imperceptible distances, the tiny (moral) differences between each step add up to a significant moral difference between propositions p and t: between the top of the slope and the bottom.

The empirical form of slippery slope argument may, or may not, be fallacious. An opponent of the legalization of voluntary euthanasia might argue that if we allow doctors to carry out acts of euthanasia, then, as a matter of fact, in the real world, this will lead to acts of non-voluntary euthanasia (and beyond). Such an opponent might accept that there is no *logical* necessity to slip from the one to the other, but that in practice such slippage will occur. Therefore, we should, as a matter of policy, not legitimate voluntary euthanasia even if such euthanasia is not, in principle, wrong.

This empirical form of argument depends on making assumptions about how the world actually is (particularly with regards to human psychology) and therefore raises the question of how compelling is the evidence for such assumptions. What in practice will happen will often depend on how precisely the policy is worded, or enforced.

The possible responses to an empirical slippery slope are threefold. First, to examine and assess the evidence that the presumed slippage will occur. Second, to consider whether there are any conceptually robust 'barriers' that can be erected to prevent slippage down the slope (e.g. the distinction between *voluntary* and *involuntary* euthanasia may provide the basis for such a barrier). Third, to consider whether any arbitrary barriers can prevent slippage (as are often used in legal settings, for example when there is an age cut-off below which a person may not legally consume alcohol) (see Figure 3).

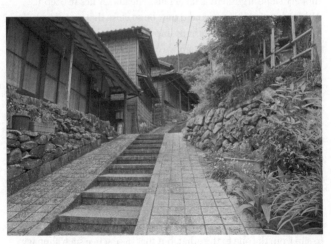

3. Slippery slope.

The slippery slope argument could be used to argue against the legalization of voluntary euthanasia (see discussion of Dr Cox in Box 3, Chapter 2) on the grounds that allowing killing in that case would inevitably lead to allowing killing in situations where it would be wrong. The validity of such an argument would depend on the evidence that such 'slippage' would in fact occur however the law was framed and however the practice was regulated.

Beyond the tools

Ethical reasoning cannot be reduced to algorithms. Situations are complex and doing the right thing will often require flexibility. Rationality, if practised in isolation from other virtues, can, like bureaucracy, become rigid and inhuman. Humane medicine will require in addition to rationality: wisdom, imagination, and creativity.

Wisdom

The motto of the Royal College of Psychiatrists, in London, is 'Let Wisdom Guide'. Wisdom, we take it, requires, at root, the combination of moral integrity with an almost intuitive grasp of the likely outcomes of our actions. It involves an understanding of how people are likely to react to a situation. In medicine it might involve a good grasp of how this particular patient, and this patient's condition, will respond to different management strategies. The wise person, most of the time, does the right thing with the right consequences. Less wise people might try to do the right thing but, too often, through poor judgement of the consequences of their actions, bring about bad outcomes. Often this will be through a misreading of how others will respond. The gaining of wisdom requires experience—a now underrated value in the wake of the emphasis on 'objective' evidence—experience gained through curiosity and reflection.

Imagination

However good our analytic abilities, our logical arguments, and our persuasive powers, we may make the wrong decisions through a lack of imagination. Imagination is needed in medicine in order to understand the perspectives and the emotions of patients, of their families, and of other members of the healthcare team. The arts and literature can help us to enlarge our imaginations and understand the range of human experience. The Latin playwright Terence wrote: 'Nothing human is alien to me'. Not a bad aspiration for the young health professional.

Creativity

We have seen that ethical argument requires creativity—creativity in developing arguments, in considering possible counter-examples, and in imagining cases for comparisons and for thought experiments. Medical ethics is about good *practice*: judging what is the right decision, the right thing to do, in a particular situation. We can at first think that the decision will be either to do *this* or to do *that*. It may take an act of creation to see that there is another possibility, perhaps one that side-steps an ethical dilemma or is better for some other reason. 'Is there another approach?' is usually a useful question to ask.

In Chapters 2 and 3 we have focused on the *techniques* of medical ethics. Socrates, one of the founders of ethics in the Western world, used his philosophical techniques to be an intellectual gadfly irritating the status quo with awkward questions and arguments. In Chapters 4 and 5 we will see how medical ethics can keep alive that valuable role for philosophical reasoning.

Chapter 4
People who don't exist; at least not yet

Medical ethics, as Chapters 2 and 3 have highlighted, is about dissecting an issue and making an argument. There is method; there are tools. But what *purposes* does it serve?

In this chapter and Chapter 5, we will see medical ethics—at its most critical—as arguing that there is something significantly wrong with how we conventionally see things. This is medical ethics challenging the status quo, making life difficult for professionals and policy-makers. Medical ethics as gadfly.

In Chapters 6 and 7, we will see medical ethics in a more coming-on disposition, giving support to those who are puzzled and uncertain of what to do. In the final section, Chapters 8 and 9, it is medical ethics itself that will be under attack.

Medicine, in general, is concerned with people who exist. But not always so. The story of medicine begins before conception. In Laurence Sterne's great novel, the eponymous hero, Tristram Shandy, suggests that a person's character, and the life he will enjoy, is shaped by his parents' thoughts during copulation. Tristram complains:

> I wish either my father or my mother, or indeed both of them, as
> they were in duty both equally bound to it, had minded what they

were about when they begot me; had they duly consider'd how much depended upon what they were then doing;—that not only the production of a rational Being was concerned in it; but that possibly the happy formation and temperature of his body, perhaps his genius and the very cast of his mind:—and, for aught they knew to the contrary, even the fortunes of his whole house might take their turn from the humours and dispositions which were then uppermost... *Pray, my Dear*, quoth my mother, *have you not forgot to wind up the clock?—Good G--!* cried my father, making an exclamation, but taking care to moderate his voice at the same time,—*Did ever woman, since the creation of the world, interrupt a man with such a silly question?*.

The Human Fertilisation and Embryology Act (HFEA)—the law that governs assisted reproduction services in the UK—requires doctors to mind what they are about when they help a woman to conceive a child. The Act imposes a duty on fertility clinics 'to consider the welfare of any child who may be born as a result of the treatment (including the need of that child for supportive parenting)'. In the original Act (1990) the words in brackets were: 'including the need of that child for a father', but this was changed to the current wording in 2008, after long Parliamentary debate. The change was made principally in light of changes in social attitudes towards single mothers and same sex partnerships. The debate was disappointing, however, because it took little or no account of a fundamental issue in the welfare considerations of 'any child who may be born': the issue known as *the non-identity problem*.

The moral implications of the non-identity problem were first discussed in detail by the British philosopher, Derek Parfit, in his book *Reasons and Persons*. These implications were largely ignored when a post-menopausal British woman aged 59 went to a private fertility clinic in Italy to be helped to conceive a child (in fact she subsequently gave birth to twins). 'Think of the poor children who will be born' was one response 'they will be the laughing stock of their friends when they are met at the school gate by such an elderly mother'. Many believe that concern for the welfare of potential children rules out fertility treatment for elderly women. To understand the non-identity problem, and why this view is wrong, let us first consider the analogy between assisted reproduction and adoption.

The analogy with adoption

In the early days of '*in vitro* fertilisation' (IVF), a Manchester woman was removed from the IVF waiting list when it was discovered that she had a criminal record involving prostitution offences. The hospital concerned had a policy in place (this was a few years before the HFEA was enacted). This policy stated that couples wanting IVF 'must in the ordinary course of events, satisfy the general criteria established by adoption societies in assessing suitability for adoption' (Kennedy and Grubb, 2000). In effect this policy meant that if a woman seeking IVF would not have been considered suitable as an adoptive parent, she should not be provided with assistance to reproduce. The underlying grounds for this policy, presumably, are the welfare of the child who would exist were fertility treatment to be given. But does this analogy between adoption and assisting reproduction hold?

In the case of adoption we have a baby (baby 'x') and a number of possible adoptive parents: A, B, C, etc. (see Figure 4).

Suppose that we have good reason to believe that parents A will be better parents than B, C, etc., and that baby 'x' is likely to have a better life if we choose parents A than if we choose any of the other parents (B, C, etc.). Assuming that judgements about the likely quality of parenting can be made (and such judgements have to be made by adoption agencies) then we act, as far as we can judge, in the best interests of baby 'x' in giving baby 'x' to parents A.

Now compare this situation of adoption with that of assisting reproduction. Suppose that couples A, B, C, etc., come for help

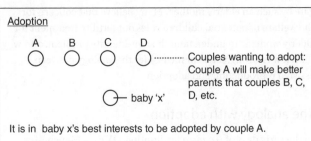

Adoption

A   B   C   D

Couples wanting to adopt: Couple A will make better parents that couples B, C, D, etc.

baby 'x'

It is in baby x's best interests to be adopted by couple A.

Assisted reproduction

A   B   C   D

Couples wanting to be helped: Couple A will make better parents that couples B, C, D, ect.

a   b   c   d

The babies who will exist if we help A, B, etc.

If we help couple B, baby b will be born. If we help couple A, baby a will be born. Baby a is a different person from baby b.

4. Adoption vs assisted reproduction.

with fertility treatment. All these couples are likely to be decent parents but we have good reason to believe that couple A are likely to be better parents than couples B, C, etc. Which couple should we help? Surely we would be acting in the best interests of the baby who may come to exist if we helped parents A, on the grounds that, as far as we can judge, the baby would have a better life with couple A than with couples B, C, etc.?

It is not, however, as simple as this. There is no kingdom, as far as we are aware, of potential babies waiting to be allocated to a particular set of parents. If we help couple A to conceive, then one baby (baby *a*) will come into existence. If we help couple B then a different baby (baby *b*) will come into existence. What sense can we make of assessing the interests of the baby that may exist at a later time? If we help couple B then baby *b* would come to exist and have a good start in life but not as good a start as baby *a* would have had. If we have the resources to help only one couple, which couple should we choose, if our only criterion is what is in the best interests of the baby who will come to exist? It is tempting to say that the best interests of the baby would be served by helping couple A. But this is wrong. It will be a different baby depending on which couple we help. It is in potential baby *a*'s best interests for us to help couple A, but in potential baby *b*'s best interests to help couple B. If we focus on the interests of the baby who may exist at a later date the question that needs to be asked is: *are these interests better served if she is born to these parents or if she never exists at all*? The question, put this way, is of course rather odd since it asks us to compare existence with non-existence. Perhaps a better question is: if there were later to exist a baby to this couple, would that baby have a reasonable expectation of a life worth living? The key is that the possibility of 'this' potential baby being born to any other (possibly better) parents does not arise. This, crucially, is where the analogy with adoption breaks down.

If we have the resources to help only one couple then an argument could be made for choosing to help couple A. The argument is as follows: if we help couple A then the baby that will exist (baby *a*) will have a better life (on the best prediction) than the baby (*b*) who would have existed had we helped couple B. If there are no other relevant grounds for choosing between the various couples then it is better to act in such a way as to bring about the existence of those babies who are likely to enjoy the best life. We are, in this case, most likely to bring about the existence of the baby who will enjoy the best life by helping couple A rather than couples B, C, etc. We should, therefore, help couple A. In choosing to help couple A we are acting *against* the best interests of the baby who would have existed in the future had we helped couple B instead. Our choice to help couple A is not on the grounds of an individual's best interests but in order to make the world a better place through choosing the couple whose baby is likely to have the best life.

This point can be made more clearly by considering the following analogy. Suppose that a hospital delays the admission of a patient who requires non-urgent surgery in order to admit a patient requiring an urgent operation. No one would maintain that it was in the best interests of the first patient that his surgery be delayed. On the contrary, it is against his best interests. The justification for acting against *his* best interests is in order to benefit the patient who needs urgent surgery. Since a choice has to be made, the decision to give priority to the patient in more urgent need seems the right one.

We seem to have found an argument that justifies the initial intuition that, in the case of assisting reproduction, we should help couple A rather than couples B, C, etc. (assuming that we have the resources to help only one couple). This argument, however, is not based on the idea of acting in the best interests of the baby who may be born. It is based, instead, on the idea of a type of welfare maximization: that is, in choosing which couple to help, we should choose the couple whose baby is likely to enjoy the best life. Does it matter that the reasons are different, if the decision is the same? The answer is that it does.

Comparing existence with non-existence

We have been assuming that we can help only one of the couples A, B, C, etc. But often this is not the case. The 59-year-old woman who went to Italy and conceived twins bore the costs herself. The clinic did not have to choose between her and someone else. The outcry in the British press was not on the grounds that some other couple would not receive help as a result of her being assisted to conceive. The outcry was on the grounds that it was against the interests of the potential child (i.e. any child who might be born) that she be helped to conceive at all.

If we focus solely on the interests of the potential child, the question, we have suggested, that needs to be asked is: are the interests of this potential child better served if she is born to these parents, or if she never exists at all? But this is a very strange question. Does it make any sense to compare existence (in whatever state) with non-existence? Some have called such a comparison as like dividing by zero—it appears to make sense at first sight, but it is a function without meaning. Others think that as long as the child will not have an appalling life then it is in the child's best interests to exist, on the grounds that, on the whole, existence is a positive thing. Perhaps some, like Montesquieu, who wrote that men [*sic*] should be mourned at their birth and not at their death ('Il faut pleurer les hommes a leur naissance, et non pas a leur mort'), take the opposite view and see existence, on balance, as a negative experience.

If those who say that one cannot compare existence with non-existence are correct then considering the best interests of children yet to be brought into existence is meaningless. But this view faces a difficulty. Let us suppose, for the sake of argument, that were couple J to have a child, that child would suffer immensely (perhaps from some dreadful genetic condition). The child would live in constant pain and finally die at the age of 1. So the life of this child would be one year of constant pain followed by death. In these circumstances it does seem to make sense to say that it would be wrong to help couple J conceive such a child on the grounds that to do so would be against the interests of the child who would exist, were we to help them.

It may be possible to make sense of this judgement without having to 'divide by zero'. Over any period of life one can ask whether, overall, the experiences are positive or negative. The zero line here is such that life above zero is overall worth living for the person concerned and life below zero is not worth living. In the case of the child who would be born to couple J, his life, overall, would rate as below zero. It is for this reason that we can say that it is in his best interests not to be born. In saying this, we do not rely on the problematic comparison of non-existence with existence, but on being able to make a judgement as to whether the life it is predicted that he would have would, overall, be above or below zero.

The argument that the post-menopausal 59-year-old woman should not be helped to conceive, on the grounds that to do so would be against the best interests of the potential child, falls apart, whichever view you take on this issue. If it makes no sense to compare existence with non-existence then it makes no sense to argue that in helping the woman conceive one is acting against the best interests of the child who does not yet exist. For on this view one cannot argue anything on the basis of best interests, since it is meaningless to compare the interests in not existing with the interests in existing. If, on the other hand, it does make sense to judge whether it is in the interests of a child (who may exist in the future) to exist, and if that judgement is essentially whether the predicted life will be, overall, a positive experience, then the question to be asked is this: is the predicted life of a child born to this 59-year-old woman, overall, likely to be positive?

Being teased at school for having an elderly mother might make a child unhappy but, unless you agree with Montesquieu, it hardly justifies the claim that overall the child's life would not be worth living. Where courts have had to decide whether it might be in the best interests of children to be allowed to die rather than have life-extending treatment, they have set the standards very high: that is, the life has to be very bad indeed for the courts to decide that it would be in the child's best interests to be allowed to die. The prospect of being teased at the school gate would not even begin to count in favour of being allowed to die. The outcry against helping the post-menopausal woman to conceive was based on the grounds that the life of the child who may exist as a result of the treatment would not go as well as that of children born to a younger mother. But that, as we have argued, is not relevant since the child born to this post-menopausal woman could not exist as the child of a younger woman.

Identity-preserving actions and identity-affecting actions

There is a fundamental distinction that arises from this discussion and that is at the heart of the non-identity problem: that between an identity-preserving and an identity-affecting action or decision.

An example of an identity-preserving action is when a pregnant woman drinks large amounts of alcohol. The drinking of the alcohol in this example does not affect the *identity* of the foetus. If the child is subsequently born with some brain damage as a result of the mother's alcohol intake that child has been harmed by the alcohol intake.

An example of an identity-affecting action is when a woman delays reproduction from, for example, 30 to 40 years of age. A different child will be born as a result of her delay. When a doctor chooses to help couple A to conceive, rather than couple B, she is making an identity-affecting decision.

In Box 8, we give some further medical situations in which the non-identity problem arises—situations in which the actions are

---

Box 8 Three clinical examples that involve the non-identity problem

1. Preimplantation genetic testing

Hypothetical case 1: 'deafening' an embryo

A couple with a genetic condition causing deafness wish to have a child who is also deaf. This is so that the child is part of the 'deaf community'. The woman becomes pregnant. Genetic testing shows that the foetus does not have the gene causing deafness: she is likely to become a normal child. Suppose that

(continued)

Box 8 Continued

a drug is available that if taken by a pregnant woman will cause a normal foetus to become deaf. It has no other effect and is otherwise completely safe for both embryo and mother.

The couple decide that the woman should take this drug in order to ensure that their child is born deaf.

a) Would the couple be morally wrong to choose to take the drug?

b) Would a doctor be wrong to prescribe the drug at the couple's request?

c) If the parents did take the drug and their child were born deaf, would the child have a morally legitimate grievance against the parents and/or the doctors?

Now consider the following hypothetical case.

Hypothetical case 2: choosing a 'deaf embryo'

A couple with a genetic condition causing deafness wish help with conceiving. A number of embryos are created, using IVF, and these are genetically tested to see which have the 'deafness gene'. Embryo A is a genetically normal embryo. Embryo B has the 'deafness gene' but is otherwise genetically normal. The couple choose to have embryo B implanted and subsequently give birth to a deaf child: child B.

If you consider that the embryo has the full moral status of a person, vary the example to involve egg, rather than embryo, selection.

a) Are the couple morally wrong to choose, for implantation, embryo B rather than embryo A?

b) Would doctors be acting wrongly to accede to their request?

c) Does child B have a morally legitimate grievance against the parents and/or the doctors?

How do your answers to the questions in cases 1 and 2 compare? At first sight it may seem wrong for the couple to choose to have a deaf child when they could have had a child with normal hearing, and wrong for doctors to allow such a choice. The principal reason why this seems wrong is that such a choice would be harmful to the child. But this is false: it is not harmful to the child because the choice of which embryo to implant is an identity-affecting choice (see main text).

2. Delaying pregnancy

A 35-year-old woman hopes in the long run to become a mother, but not yet. She wants to delay pregnancy for another four years until she has finished a degree course. She knows that she is more likely to conceive a child with trisomy 21 (Down syndrome) if she delays pregnancy. She asks her doctor for a prescription for the contraceptive pill. The doctor prescribes the pill for the next three and a half years. After this the woman becomes pregnant and has a child with trisomy 21. Did the doctor's act, in prescribing the contraceptive pill, harm the child? No. It would have been a different child who was born had the doctor not prescribed the pill.

3. Treating acne

Acne is a skin condition that typically affects adolescents. It is characterized by spots and small pustules that are distributed over the face. Very severe acne, if left untreated, can lead not only to psychological problems but also to permanent facial scarring. Sometimes the only effective treatment is a drug called isotretinoin. There is one, very important, unwanted effect of isotretinoin: it may cause foetal damage if a woman is taking the treatment during pregnancy. Children may be born with congenital malformations mainly of facial appearance or of the heart.

(continued)

Box 8 Continued

Because of the significance of these unwanted effects on a foetus it would normally be considered wrong for a doctor to prescribe isotretinoin to a woman with severe acne known to be pregnant, even if the woman wanted the treatment, because of the harm to the foetus, or at any rate to the child that the foetus will become.

What should a doctor do, however, in circumstances where a patient is not pregnant, but might become so while taking the drug? The advice that is given to doctors is that they should prescribe the isotretinoin only if the woman will reliably delay pregnancy until after she has stopped taking the isotretinoin. In some situations this will require the doctor to prescribe the isotretinoin only in combination with the contraceptive pill.

On this view it is right for a doctor to prescribe isotretinoin to a non-pregnant woman if she will reliably delay pregnancy until after the course of isotretinoin (typically six months to a year); but wrong to prescribe it if she will not reliably delay pregnancy. The intuition is that if she does not delay pregnancy, and the child is born with congenital malformations, then she has harmed the child, but if she does delay pregnancy then she has not harmed the child. Once again, however, it will be a different child: it cannot be claimed that the child has been harmed as a result of the woman's not delaying pregnancy. For if the woman had delayed pregnancy that child would not have existed at all. However, it can be said that the child has been harmed by the woman taking isotretinoin.

identity-affecting. In all these cases it can certainly be argued that it would be better if the decision were made that would lead to the birth of whichever child would be likely to have the better life. Such an argument could be based on the idea of maximizing overall welfare, as we outlined previously. In none of the cases given in Box 8, however, can an argument be based on the interests of the potential child. Neither can it be claimed, whichever decision is made, that the child born has been harmed by the decision.

The non-identity issue has an important impact on what doctors should do. Where the doctor aids an act—such as in prescribing a drug during pregnancy that may harm the foetus—then such harm provides a good reason for the doctor to refuse to prescribe the drug. Prescribing the drug is an example of an identity-preserving action. But when the doctor's action is an identity-affecting action that may lead to a child being born disabled or diseased in some way then there is no child who has been made worse off than he could otherwise have been. In societies that give considerable weight both to patient autonomy and reproductive choice, doctors should not normally override a woman's choice in situations where no person is harmed; and, in identity-affecting decisions or acts, no person is harmed (unless the child's life, overall, would not be worth living). Such a conclusion suggests that it is almost always wrong for doctors, or society more generally, to refuse reproductive assistance on grounds of the welfare of the potential child. This conclusion goes against normal intuition. In this case, it seems to us, normal intuition is wrong: it is based on a false metaphysics.

Chapter 5
Inconsistencies about madness

The problem we will discuss in this chapter is not metaphysical but political. It is an issue of justice. The gadfly of medical ethics will probe the rationale for the laws and policies that impact on those suffering from mental illness, and find them wanting. But first we raise an even more profound difficulty. The very question of what should count as mental illness is burdened with political and social prejudices.

In 1851, Dr Samuel Cartwright published an article in a New Orleans medical journal describing the mental illness of drapetomania, an illness from which black slaves suffered and manifest by a tendency to run away from their white masters.

In 1952, the first edition of the US *Diagnostic and Statistical Manual of Mental Disorders* was published. Homosexuality was listed as a mental disorder and its status was confirmed in 1968. In 1973, the American Psychiatric Association voted, by a small margin, to remove homosexuality from the list of mental disorders.

The classificatory system of disease that is used in most of Europe is the *International Classification of Diseases* published by the World Health Organisation. The current edition includes fetishism as a mental disorder. This is described as: 'Reliance

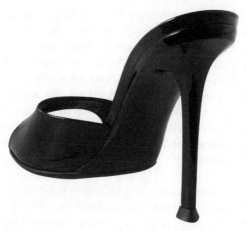

5. High-heeled shoe.

on some non-living object as stimulus for sexual arousal and sexual gratification...such as articles of clothing or footwear' (Figure 5). Will fetishism still be classified as a mental disorder in twenty years' time? Should it be?

The example of homosexuality shows that adopting a policy that allows people to be treated medically even with their full consent can be ethically problematic. Two generations ago people would voluntarily seek 'treatment' for their homosexuality. Medicine offered the possibility of altering sexual orientation. We would now consider it wrong that society expected medical practitioners to be complicit with this practice. Social attitudes, not illness, were the problem—and these attitudes can become particularly pernicious when they are written into policy documents and laws that govern treatment. What is to count as mental illness can be ethically problematic even in the context of voluntary treatment.

Psychiatry, unlike most branches of medicine, is given the authority to sometimes impose treatment on people against their will. Some argue that this is necessarily wrong, but one has only to see the distress that people with untreated schizophrenia can experience to question such a position. Mental illness can affect the person's understanding such that he does not see that he is ill and will benefit from treatment. Most liberal democracies have formal procedures allowing psychiatrists this power to enforce treatment, and for humane reasons. As the example of drapetomania shows, this power can be abused, and has been abused by repressive regimes, in diagnosing political dissent as mental disorder.

People with mental disorder may be securely detained against their will not only for treatment but also for the safety of others. Again this practice is often humane. Many of us would want to be detained in order to be prevented from being violent to others if we were to suffer a mental disorder that involved, for example, the delusion that we were being attacked. A psychiatric hospital seems a more appropriate place than a prison for such detention. Again, however, such practice is open to abuse, and not only in repressive societies. In this chapter we will argue that those with mental disorder, even in liberal democracies, are subject to a double injustice as a result of current policy.

Crime and mental illness

It is the criminal law that deals mainly with situations where one person harms another. In English law, and that of many other countries, for a person to be guilty of a crime it must be proven that it was this person who carried out the relevant act; *and* that this person had the state of mind necessary to be held responsible for that act. The first aspect is called the *actus reus* ('guilty act') and the second the *mens rea* ('guilty mind').

A person who suffers from a mental illness and commits what could have been regarded as a criminal act may be found 'not guilty' because, due to the illness, she is not responsible for her behaviour. Crudely put: her body committed the act, but her mind did not commit the crime.

A key English case was that of Daniel McNaughten who suffered the delusional belief, among others, that the Tory Party was plotting to murder him. He decided to kill its leader, Robert Peel. In 1843, he shot Peel's secretary but was prevented from firing a second shot. McNaughten was acquitted of murder on the grounds of insanity and was sent to a secure psychiatric hospital. The case led to the drawing up of the rules (the 'McNaughten rules') for determining when someone should be considered 'not guilty' on grounds of insanity.

Protecting society from dangerous people

A person without mental disorder who commits a violent crime of sufficient gravity is typically sent to prison in part as retribution (he deserves to be punished) and in part to protect society.

There are two crucial liberal principles that are incorporated into criminal law—and are part of the European Convention on Human Rights:

1. A person who has not (yet) committed a crime cannot be detained on the grounds that it is expected that she will commit a crime.
2. A person must be allowed back into the community once he has served his prison sentence, although some crimes may attract a life sentence.

We will use the term 'preventive detention' to refer to keeping someone in a secure environment (prison or a secure psychiatric hospital) on grounds of protection of others in one, or both, of the following situations: when the person has not (yet) committed a violent act; and when she has committed such an act and been in a secure environment for the length of the prison sentence appropriate to the act. These two liberal principles can be re-written as: 'A person cannot be preventively detained'. Special sentences that link the length of imprisonment with ongoing assessments of risk that the person poses to the public have been attempted, but these have not stood the test of time and are widely seen to be unjust.

The recognition in policy circles of this injustice does not, however, extend to people with a mental disorder. If you have committed a violent act as a result of mental illness you can be detained in a psychiatric hospital for as long as it is thought that you pose sufficient risk to others. This may well be much longer than a criminal without a diagnosed mental disorder would be detained in prison for a similar violent act. Indeed, if you suffer a mental disorder you may be so detained on the grounds that you might be dangerous even if you have not yet committed a violent act. What worries us is the inequity in treatment between those with, and those without, a diagnosed mental disorder.

There is, of course, an important issue of public policy as to how society should protect itself against people who pose significant risk of harm to others. The argument we want to make is about consistency. If two people, A who is mentally ill and B who is not mentally ill, pose the same risk of harm to others then, if it is right to preventatively detain A (on grounds of this risk of harm) it is right to do so to B. Conversely if it is wrong to preventatively detain B (as European legislation states) then it is wrong to detain A. Otherwise we are discriminating against the mentally ill.

Are there any reasons that justify such apparent discrimination? We can think of four, but none, in our opinion, justifies a different approach to preventive detention.

1. The mentally ill person is more dangerous.
2. The assessment of risk of harm is more certain in the case of those with mental illness.

3. It may be the case that prolonging detention in hospital will lead to further improvement in the mental illness, and further reduction in risk of harm, to others. It would be an error to release the patient from the secure psychiatric hospital when a further period in hospital would reduce risk.

4. There is a distinction between what a person wants when mentally ill and what the person would want if cured of the mental illness. It is typically the case that those mentally ill patients who are preventively detained remain chronically ill. That is why they remain at risk of harming others, and why they continue to be detained. It is possible, at least in theory, to distinguish between what the ill person wants, and what the person might have wanted if well. It is also reasonable to say that his *genuine* wishes are those he would have when well, and that his genuine wishes would be to remain preventively detained, if he continued to be ill and a danger to others. Respecting the authentic wishes and autonomy of the person when well would mean preventively detaining the person when ill (and dangerous).

We will consider each of these four reasons in turn.

The first reason is irrelevant. The situation we are considering is where the two people—the person with and the person without the diagnosed mental illness—pose the same risk of harm to others. Indeed, the law in England does not permit preventive detention for dangerous people without diagnosed mental disorder in any circumstance.

The second reason might provide weak grounds for a difference in approach if it were true—but it is not. Assessment of risk of harm to others is notoriously difficult whether we are dealing with mentally disordered people or not. In any case, the point at issue is whether risk of harm justifies preventive detention. The level of uncertainty over the estimation of risk might alter the threshold but not the principle of preventive detention.

The third reason does not provide grounds for treating those with mental illness differently from those without. In both cases a detained person might pose less of a risk of harm to others if further detained. If this continuing reduction in risk gives grounds for preventive detention in those with mental illness then it also provides grounds for preventive detention of those without.

The fourth reason provides the best argument but even this is unconvincing. The distinction between what a person wants when mentally ill and what she wants when well might be made if the person's views when well can be ascertained. But many of the mentally ill people who are violent are either those with chronic mental illness or those with a personality disorder. In neither case is it likely that we have good evidence about their 'authentic wishes'—their wishes when well. Furthermore there is no good reason to expect, in these settings, that the person would wish to be detained and to lead a life of very limited freedoms. In the absence of such evidence it seems highly dubious to keep the person detained on the grounds of respecting his autonomy.

We conclude that if we think it right for society to preventively detain mentally ill people who present a certain level of risk of harm to others then we should do the same for those who are not mentally ill. Conversely if we think preventive detention is an unacceptable infringement of human rights in the case of people without mental illness, it is an unacceptable infringement of human rights for those with mental illness. We leave open which way we ought to go. The point we want to make is that the current position is untenable because it is inconsistent and unjust. Policy must change accordingly.

Enforcing treatment for the sake of the mentally ill person

The *double* injustice referred to earlier in this chapter is that those with mental disorder are not only discriminated against for the protection of others but also for the protection of themselves.

It is a long-standing principle in medical ethics and law that those who are ill, but retain the mental capacity to make a decision, may refuse beneficial, even life-saving, treatment. A classic example is when a Jehovah's witness refuses blood transfusion even if she is likely to die without the transfusion. This principle applies to the treatment of physical illness. It does not apply, however, in many countries, including the UK, to those with mental illness. For example, under the English Mental Health Act a person who has a mental disorder may be treated for his mental disorder despite refusal even if he retains the mental capacity to refuse consent. This is unjust unless it were true that anyone with a mental disorder is *ipso facto* lacking the mental capacity to refuse treatment. But it is not true. Some people with a mental disorder will lack decision-making capacity. Some won't. It may be right to impose life-saving treatment on a patient who has the capacity to refuse treatment or it may be wrong. But what is not right is to change the answer according to whether or not the person has a mental disorder. To do so is to discriminate, once again, against those suffering from a mental illness. Again, policy must change accordingly.

Chapter 6
Helping the helper

Chapters 4 and 5 may have given the impression that those who work in medical ethics are a rather troublesome group. By picking at arguments, prodding at inconsistencies, and pouncing on specific words, they are unlikely to endear themselves to healthcare professionals or policy-makers. It might be grudgingly accepted that such gadflies, such critics of the status quo, serve a useful purpose, but they would hardly be welcomed, one would think, onto a hospital ward. Socrates, the original philosopher-gadfly, was, after all, put to death by the Athenian state.

In this chapter, and Chapter 7, we will see ethics playing a rather different role: that of support to harassed healthcarers and puzzled policy-makers. There is an analogy here with the role that *evidence-based medicine* has played in recent years. The requirement to provide evidence-based medicine has meant that doctors and medical researchers have been challenged to provide clear evidence on which to base, and justify, clinical decisions. But, although this requirement has led to challenges to the status quo, it has also provided support to clinicians through a clarification of the criteria for assessing good scientific evidence, and in enabling such evidence to be gathered. There remain, however, many clinical situations in which the scientifically right decision is not clear. One treatment may have some advantages over another while also presenting disadvantages. Furthermore it can be difficult to predict, despite the results from large clinical trials, how a particular patient will respond to a given treatment. There is not necessarily one right answer—one best treatment—but, to the good clinician, it is still important that the decision made, whatever it is, be made after reasoned consideration of the relevant issues and evidence. Furthermore, the good clinician will want to be able to properly justify the decision made. In this situation the clinician might be assisted by the use of expertise in pharmacology or physiology, or that in the assessment of evidence. The clinician may have acquired the expertise herself or she might seek the advice and support of someone else with such expertise.

As it is for the scientific aspects of healthcare, so it is with the ethical aspects. When a situation is ethically complex, when there are ethical grounds in support of differing approaches to patient care, good healthcare professionals will wish to ensure that the decisions are taken only after proper consideration. Some expertise in medical ethics will be necessary. They may themselves have such expertise or they may seek the support of someone with such expertise: another caregiver or a medical ethicist—that is, someone with special training in the ethical aspects of healthcare.

In this chapter we show how ethics support can be introduced to shape ethical understanding and good care practice. We have chosen an example from a context outside a specifically medical setting, a setting that has not typically been subject to the ethicist's gaze: the everyday care provided to people with dementia in care homes. This is deliberate. As more and more people are living into old age, the world over, so dementia—a condition that increases in prevalence with age—is becoming more common. The question of how to care for people with dementia, and of how to cope with the ethical problems that arise in providing day-to-day support to them, is urgent. Medical ethics includes, in our view, coverage of ethical issues that arise for carers as a result of illness and disease. Indeed doctors, and other health professionals, can become involved in all aspects of the care of people with chronic disease. Focusing only on those issues that are recognizably part of providing healthcare to people with dementia is to risk making invisible the common, everyday challenges of those who struggle to address them.

The medical ethicist on call

In some hospitals, particularly in the United States, providing ethics support has become a professionalized activity. Medical ethics consultants are employed by healthcare providers and are available, on call, to consult on ethical problems as they arise in patient care. In the UK, medical ethicists are rarely employed in these professional roles, and instead, serve as members of clinical ethics committees or advisory groups that are convened within a health or care setting. These committees, typically made up of a mix of different care professionals, consider specific cases that those working in the hospital or community are finding ethically problematic.

In modern healthcare practice, the multi-disciplinary team is crucial to ensuring the optimal management of patient care. It plays a pivotal role in providing a supportive environment to share and resolve ethical problems. Opposing points of views between team members can be identified and potential difficulties in carrying out an ethically robust decision ironed out. But sometimes there will be such significant disagreement between team members that agreeing the ethically right decision will appear impossible. Other times, decisions need to be made that are particularly serious or significant. On these occasions, medical ethicists may be called in to team meetings or ward rounds, to offer ethics input—the ethicist becomes part of the team that makes the clinical decisions. One care home was faced with the following situation.

The case of the poppy-wearing conscientious objector

A staff member, Anne, described what had happened:

It was close to Remembrance Sunday—the day in November that commemorates the contribution of British and Commonwealth servicemen and -women in the two world wars and subsequent conflicts. A war veteran had visited the care home selling poppies, the flower traditionally worn to mark the occasion (Figure 6). Poppies were given to each resident. The staff decided to organize an activity for the residents in the main lounge on Sunday morning including watching the Remembrance Sunday service on TV. The staff knew that three of the residents had fought in the war, and thought that this event would be appreciated by all.

On the Friday before the service, however, the daughter of Mr Andrews, one of the residents, visited her father and was

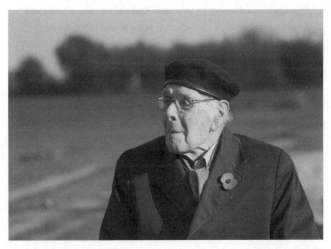

6. Remembrance poppy.

shocked to see him wearing a poppy on his jacket lapel. Mr Andrews' daughter told Anne that her father had been a conscientious objector all his life. He would have been mortified, his daughter said, if he had known, prior to getting dementia, that he would end up in a care home wearing a poppy and watching a Remembrance Sunday service.

Anne removed Mr Andrews' poppy and told other members of staff that he was not to join in the group activity on Sunday. She felt that this was the appropriate way of treating Mr Andrews with respect.

On the Sunday morning, however, another member of staff gave Mr Andrews a new poppy, and encouraged him to join in watching the Remembrance Sunday service. When Anne realized what was happening, she removed Mr Andrews' poppy and led him out of the lounge. Mr Andrews became upset. He attempted to grab the poppy from Anne and to walk back into the lounge.

Other members of staff at the time had strongly expressed their view that Anne had acted wrongly in causing Mr Andrews distress in this way. Since then, Anne had slept badly worrying about whether or not she had acted correctly.

This case is one example of an ethical issue that arises frequently in the care of people with dementia: how to balance the person's previous preferences and values with their current interests, when these conflict. This issue can take different forms, depending on the specific circumstances. For example, the question might be whether to respect a person with dementia's previous commitment to vegetarianism; or whether it is ethically right to prevent two men with dementia engaging in mutual sexual touching, when this touching appears to give both men pleasure but when both men have identified as being heterosexual previously. Further examples of ethically problematic situations that arise in the everyday care of people with dementia are given in Box 9.

Box 9 Some ethically problematic situations that arise in the care of people with dementia

Balancing freedoms and risks

People with dementia may be at risk in several ways. They may wander out into the street and get lost, and be at risk from traffic or from hypothermia. They may be in danger from eating inappropriately stored food or from misusing electrical appliances. To what extent should we restrict a person's freedom (e.g. lock her in her house) or use surveillance devices, or take her from her own home into a care home in order to minimize risks?

Balancing the interests of various people

Allowing one person freedom may interfere with the interests of other residents or patients. Some people shout out almost constantly unless given some sedation. Some wander into other people's rooms. To what extent should we restrict freedom or impose sedation on one person for the sake of others.

Deception

Sometimes a person with dementia refuses all medication, spitting it out or not allowing it in his mouth in the first place. Is it ever justified to give the medication surreptitiously, for example by hiding it in food? Does it make a difference whether the medication is for diabetes, heart failure, or sedation to ensure that the person does not disturb others at night?

Lying

A person with dementia keeps forgetting that her husband is dead and frequently asks where he is. When told he has died she becomes very upset. Should the carers always, or even usually, tell her that her husband has died, or should they tell a 'white lie' (e.g. 'he will be back in an hour or two') knowing that she will have forgotten about her husband before the hour is up?

At the ethics support meeting convened to discuss this situation several issues were considered.

Issue 1:   to what extent is Mr Andrews the same person as before the onset of dementia?

After Anne had described what had happened, it was clear that her uncertainty was shared by most members of staff. One carer, Steve, suggested that, because Mr Andrews was no longer able to remember the values that he had held when he was a conscientious objector, he no longer held those values. For Steve, people change throughout their lives, and their values are relevant only in so far as they continue to endorse them as their own. According to Steve, dementia had led to a change in Mr Andrews' values and his previous conscientious objection was no longer relevant.

In response, Anne argued that it was incorrect to say that this value of conscientious objection was no longer his value. Just because he could no longer remember holding this value did not render it irrelevant. It was not the case that he had changed his mind. Steve responded that although, because of the dementia, Mr Andrews had not changed his mind, his mind had changed him. To a significant extent he was no longer the same man. The current Mr Andrews, Steve concluded, was not a conscientious objector. Anne disagreed. Although she accepted that Mr Andrews had changed in important ways since he developed dementia, nevertheless 'to everyone who knows him, Mr Andrews is still Mr Andrews. It's still the same man that we're taking care of.'

This discussion raises some difficult philosophical questions about how a person's identity should be understood when that person is cognitively impaired. At this point the medical ethicist gave a brief explanation of two accounts of personal identity relevant to the discussion (see Box 10). Steve's view looks to be close to the 'psychological continuity' account. For him, to base

Box 10 Two concepts of personal identity

There have been many different philosophical accounts of the concept of personal identity. In the setting of dementia care, two ways of conceptualizing identity have been the most influential.

1. The psychological continuity account

On this account, what it means to be the same person is the continuity that exists over time in an individual's psychological characteristics: memories, intentions, thoughts, beliefs, affective states, and dispositions. Personal identity, on this view, is the degree of connectedness of an individual's psychological characteristics over time. One implication is that over time, as we change psychologically, so our identity changes to some extent. Rather than thinking of identity as all or nothing—that I am the same person over my life-time, and you are a completely separate person—identity is seen as a matter of degree. I am, to some extent only, the same person as my 16-year-old self.

This account can perhaps best be understood by the following thought experiment (that has been the basis of many science fiction novels and films). Consider two people, person A and person B. One morning a strange transformation suddenly takes place. The person who looks like person A—the person with A's body—has all the memories, thoughts, personality, and other psychological features of person B; and vice versa. The person with A's body wakes up thinking that he is B—and gets a surprise when he looks in the mirror. Similarly the person with B's body thinks (at least until he too looks in the mirror) that she is A. The question is: who is the same person now as the person who, the day before, was person A? Many people's intuition is to answer that it is the person who has the same psychological makeup as the person who was person A—even though he is 'in' B's body. It is this intuition that gives rise to the psychological account of personal identity.

(continued)

Box 10 Continued

Derek Parfit, who extensively developed this view, recognized that it conflicts with our everyday sense of what a person is. However, he thought this liberates us from the way we typically see our journeys through life, with good consequences for us all. As he eloquently put it:

> My life seemed like a glass tunnel, through which I was moving faster every year, and at the end of which there was darkness... When I changed my view, the walls of my glass tunnel disappeared. I now live in the open air. There is still a difference between my life and the lives of other people. But the difference is less. Other people are closer. I am less concerned about the rest of my own life, and more concerned about the lives of others.

With regards to dementia care, this account implies that the changes associated with memory loss, cognitive impairment, and personality change in dementia mean that the person with dementia should be judged to be, at least to a significant extent, a different person from the person who existed before the onset of dementia.

2. The situated-embodied-agent account

On this account, which has a strong advocate in the philosopher and physician, Julian Hughes, a person's life understood as lived in relation to other people is a major determinant of personal identity. What is important is the individual's life narrative connecting the identity of a person and the person's body, with the details of the existence that this person constructs for himself, and that is constructed about that person by other people, over time.

With regards to dementia care, this account of identity implies that the onset of dementia has relatively little impact on the person's personal identity. The person continues to exist in the same body, most commonly still standing in relation to

> many of the same people who give meaning to the person's life.
> Personal identity survives even advanced dementia, with the
> condition simply being one aspect of the person's life that
> is incorporated into the narrative that we tell about ourselves
> and about other persons.

decisions on the values held by the former Mr Andrews would be to essentially hijack who Mr Andrews currently is and to treat him as though he were someone else.

Anne's response endorses the 'situated-embodied-agent' account. On her view, Mr Andrews has not changed identity. Furthermore, although he no longer remembers that he was a conscientious objector he has not rejected his previous view: he simply no longer has the cognitive ability to form a view. For her, respecting Mr Andrews includes respecting features of his life before the onset of dementia and in particular respecting the values that were important to him.

Issue 2:   even if Mr Andrews is not the same person as before, should this affect his care?

As the discussion progressed, another member of the care team, Simon, said that Mr Andrews sometimes remembers aspects of his life before the onset of dementia, and reminisces favourably about them. For Simon, this fact is significant. Anne then said that even if the psychological continuity account were right in theory, it went so far against established good policy on advanced care planning that it simply couldn't be used to guide practice without a change in how good care was thought about more generally.

These two points highlight two further reasons in support of the argument that Mr Andrews is the same person that he was before the onset of dementia.

First, the fact that Mr Andrews could remember and endorse aspects of his life before dementia meant that, even on the psychological continuity account of personhood, he was, to a significant extent, still the same person.

Second, the view that the current Mr Andrews is a different person from the former Mr Andrews to such a degree that his former values are irrelevant is at odds not only with current views on advanced care planning but also with many established laws and practices. The laws in the UK, US, and many other countries require a person's previous wishes, values, and directives to be taken into account when he loses the cognitive capacity to make his own decisions. These laws and practices may, of course, be wrong. There is, however, one problematic implication of considering the current Mr Andrews to be a different person from the Mr Andrews before dementia. That problem is that it would then seem wrong to use any of the earlier Mr Andrews' savings to make the current Mr Andrews' life more comfortable.

The group concluded that the arguments to the effect that Mr Andrews is the same person now as before the onset of dementia were the stronger arguments and that therefore Mr Andrews' previous value of conscientious objection was relevant: it provided a reason to act as Anne had done. The group identified, however, a further question: should Mr Andrews' valuing of conscientious objection throughout much of his life trump his current preferences and well-being?

Issue 3:   should Mr Andrews' current well-being take priority over his previous wishes?

Anne argued that the values that have shaped our lives over a number of years are what define us as unique individuals, and therefore that they must be given a great deal of weight in guiding the decisions made on our behalf when we get dementia. This, she said, was how people could maintain control over their life, even at a time when, because of dementia, making simple decisions can be difficult. In response, Mary, another member of staff, said that if the issue was about control, Mr Andrews should have been left to wear the poppy and remain in the lounge: Anne had been controlling him by intervening.

The discussion then turned from *control* to *well-being*.

Staff members considered whether or not Anne's behaviour had overall enhanced Mr Andrews' well-being. At this point, the medical ethicist interjected, noting that the meaning of the concept of well-being was at stake. He suggested that those who wished to prioritize previous values on the grounds of promoting well-being would have to accept that enhancing well-being would sometimes require them to knowingly cause a resident distress. All members of staff found this conclusion difficult to accept. They concluded that if maximizing well-being were the ethical priority then the right thing would have been to let Mr Andrews wear the poppy and remain in the lounge. That brought the group back to considering the weight to be given to respecting Mr Andrews' previous values.

At this point Steve proposed a new argument: although Mr Andrews has dementia this does not mean that we should ignore his current wishes or presume that the dementia prevents him from having wishes. Through his behaviour—snatching back the poppy and trying to remain in the lounge—he was clearly expressing his current wishes. For Steve, the issue was not just about balancing previous values and wishes against current well-being, it was also about balancing previous values against current wishes, and, Steve concluded, 'doesn't Mr Andrews have the right to act in light of his immediate preferences, even if these are not reasoned through?'

In the end the group came to the conclusion that minimizing Mr Andrews' distress together with respecting his current wishes as expressed by his behaviour weighed more strongly than respecting the values he had held before dementia. Despite the fact that this conclusion did not endorse Anne's behaviour, she felt supported by the group discussion since it had taken seriously the reasons in support of what she had done. The discussion led to two further practical decisions. First, that two staff members would let Mr Andrews' daughter know what had happened and also of the group discussion. Second, that this episode had highlighted that there was no effective system in place for communicating residents' previous values to all members of staff, nor for discussing how, and to what extent, to honour them. Such a system should be put in place.

The reader may or may not agree with the group's conclusion. There are good reasons in support of what Anne did as well as of what the group concluded. Ethical arguments, like scientific evidence, might reasonably lead one person to one conclusion, and another person to another conclusion. In the end, a judgement must be made. It is important, however, that health professionals and other carers, in coming to a decision, properly consider the main issues. And society, quite rightly, may hold such professionals to account, demanding reasoned justification for the decisions made and the actions taken.

Using case comparisons

In testing and reviewing the decision and the reasons for it the reader may find some case comparisons useful. Here are some examples. The reader may wish to add further cases.

1. The case as presented except that Mr Andrews, very early after the onset of dementia, had written a statement to the effect that, if he needed care, he wanted his conscientious objection to be fully respected.

2. A care home is asked by the relatives of a man with dementia to ensure that he does not eat meat as he had been vegetarian. The staff feed him only vegetarian food. At breakfast, however, when most residents are served a 'full English', he tries, and sometimes succeeds, to eat the bacon and sausages on other residents' plates, and devours them with great pleasure.

What should the staff do? Does the reason for his previous vegetarianism make a difference—for example, if it had been a moral choice based on animal welfare; a commitment based on religious belief; or on the basis simply of taste?

3. A widow, happily married for almost sixty years, has dementia and is being cared for in a care home. She starts a relationship with a man in the home in which there is some physical touching of a sexual nature. The woman's son, on realizing this, tells the staff that they must stop this relationship from developing or being physical in any way: 'my mother would have been horrified to think that she could ever have done those things with a man other than my father'. Should a member of staff intervene to prevent this new relationship from developing further, perhaps by keeping the woman and man apart?

Sometimes the sexual touching takes place between two residents of the same sex, in a situation where both residents had identified as being heterosexual throughout their lives and when they had never previously expressed any sexual preferences towards people of the same sex. Would this feature of the situation make a difference to how care staff should act? One argument behind thinking that there is an ethical difference between this situation and the first one lies in the claim that people's sexual identity (i.e. whether they identify as heterosexual, homosexual, bisexual, etc.) is a feature of these people's identities that is more essential to who they are than their choices to engage in unexpected sexual behaviours with people of the sex for which they have a consistent sexual preference.

Chapter 7
Establishing fair procedure

In January 1997, Tony Bullimore was attempting to sail round the world in the Vendée Globe race. He had reached the dangerous and cold waters of the Southern Ocean, over 1,500 miles south of the Australian coast, when his boat was capsized by hurricane force winds. He spent four days trapped under its hull before he was rescued in the largest and most expensive such operation undertaken by the Australian defence forces (Figure 7). How much money should a civilized society spend to try to save Tony Bullimore? Is the answer 'whatever it takes', or should there be a limit?

Let us pose a more general question: what is the cash value of a human life? This question is a disturbing one to ask but, paradoxically, there are situations where avoiding the question may cost lives. Determining how a society allocates scarce medical resources is one situation where this question is faced head on.

No healthcare system in the world has sufficient money to provide the best possible treatment for all patients in all situations, not even those spending large sums on healthcare. New, better, and expensive treatments are being developed all the time. When is the extra benefit worth the extra cost? All healthcare systems must address this question, whether mixed private- and

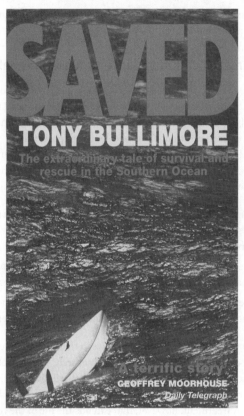

7. **Cover of *Saved*.**

insurance-based systems, such as in the US, or publicly funded
systems, such as the British National Health Service. Since the
best treatment cannot always be provided, trade-offs must
be made, healthcare must be *rationed*. Even a totally private
system rations healthcare. It does so on the basis of the person's
ability to pay, surely one of the least equitable grounds possible.
Our claim in this chapter is that medical ethics can provide,

and indeed has provided, practical support to assist policy-makers in such allocation of healthcare resources.

Resource allocation and incommensurable values

Imagine that you lead a health service for a particular population. You have a limited budget. You have decided how to spend most of your budget and you have a few hundred thousand pounds left, as yet uncommitted. There are, let us suppose, three new and improved treatments that you are not currently funding. You have the resources to fund one, but only one. Which should you choose? The possibilities are:

1. A new treatment for bowel cancer that gives patients a small but significant chance of increased life expectancy over current (cheaper) treatments.

2. A new drug that lowers the chance of death from heart attack in patients with genetically induced raised blood cholesterol.

3. A new surgical device that ensures a lower mortality than current treatment from a particularly difficult kind of brain surgery

On what basis should you choose between these possibilities? In each case some people stand to die prematurely, and in each case the treatment increases the chance that they will live for longer. As a starting point, it seems fair to value every individual's life equally. A treatment, however, that extends the life of the relevant patients by many years would seem more valuable than one that extends life by only one year. So perhaps we should value each year of life *gained*, as a result of the treatment, equally, no matter which individuals benefit. Applying this principle, the right way of spending the money available would be to 'buy' as much extra life as possible. This approach looks fair: we are valuing each unit of extra life equally, regardless of whose life it is.

We come up against a problem, however: *the distribution problem*. Take a look at the three interventions in Table 1.

Table 1 Choosing between three interventions

Intervention	How many people benefit	Total years of life gained
1	10	35
2	15	30
3	2	16

Suppose that each of these interventions costs the same and we can only afford one. Suppose further that the distributions are as follows:

- Of the ten people who are benefited by intervention 1, the average benefit is 3.5 years. The range is two to four years.
- Of the fifteen people who are benefited by intervention 2, the average benefit is two years. The range is one to three years.
- The two people who are benefited by intervention 3 will each enjoy eight more years of life.

Which of the three interventions should we choose?

If we think that what we should do is to 'buy' the maximum amount of extra life that we can (*the maximization view*) then we should put our money into intervention 1 because we buy thirty-five extra years. This is more than we will get with the other two interventions. However, you might think that intervention 2 is preferable because we help more people (fifteen as opposed to ten) although each person gains fewer extra years of life. Or, you might think that intervention 3 is the best option because the two people who are helped receive a really significant gain (eight years of life)—compared with a maximum of four years for intervention 1. This case comparison leads us to consider whether it is not only the total number of years gained that matters, but also the ways in which those years are distributed between people.

There are further grounds for rejecting the maximization view. A common intuition is that those who are very badly off—those, for example, who are very ill and in grave danger of almost immediate death—should be a higher priority than those less ill, even if the former stand to gain fewer extra years of life. This view is sometimes expressed by saying that patients should be prioritized, at least to some extent, according to their *need*. A second intuition that many people have is that those who bear responsibility for bringing an illness on themselves should be at lower priority than those who are ill through no fault of their own. A third intuition is that we might also value a year of life differently for people of different ages. For example, we might view extending the life by one year of a person aged 20 as more valuable than a similar extension of life in a person aged 80. The various values at stake here, for example maximizing the amount of extra life as against prioritizing those with the greatest need, are highly contested, and we can reasonably disagree between ourselves about the weight that should be given to these values. In any case, no matter how good the evidence about the effects of the various treatments, we cannot avoid ethical values. Science cannot solve the conflict between values: value-free evidence-based policy-making is a myth.

Medical ethics and fair procedure

We saw in Chapter 6 how medical ethics and ethicists can provide support to those involved in making difficult decisions. It is not that ethics provides 'the answer' but rather that it is a discipline that is concerned with clarifying the ethical values at stake and analysing the arguments—their strengths and weaknesses. Although there may be reasonable disagreement about which are the key values and how they are to be balanced, it is important that decisions are based on a proper consideration of the relevant values and arguments. Medical ethics can, and does, play this supporting role when decisions are made in the setting of resource allocation. We will first, however, highlight a rather different role.

The policy decisions that must be made when allocating healthcare resources impact on us all. Because of this impact, we, the general public, as recipients of healthcare resources, might reasonably claim a stake in how these decisions are made, in a way that we do not in decisions that are made within the private space of the doctor–patient relationship. In short, policy-makers need to be accountable to us in some way. This view chimes with the expectations that we have about how our social institutions should function more generally in a democratic society. Precisely how such accountability should operate is not straightforward. This is partly because the evidence needed to properly consider the values in resource allocation decisions requires a highly technical understanding of medical evidence. Furthermore, decisions need to be taken and reviewed frequently as new treatments become available.

These considerations lead us to ask a question more commonly discussed within political philosophy than ethics: not 'what is the *right decision*?' but 'what is the *right procedure* for making decisions?'

Two American ethicists, Norman Daniels and James Sabin, developed a procedural approach for fair decision-making for allocating health resources that has influenced several health policy institutions. These include the UK's National Institute for Health and Care Excellence (NICE) which makes rationing decisions in the setting of the National Health Service. The central idea is that the procedure should be *reasonable* and *accountable* to the public. In practice, where this approach has been adopted, the procedure involves at its core a group, or groups, of people who take the key decisions. The people who constitute such decision-making groups typically include: those with specific relevant *expertise* such as medical, scientific, economic, and ethics expertise; those with relevant *experience*, such as patients or those who represent patient groups; and 'lay people' who represent the general public. The composition of the group is chosen to try and ensure that the decisions taken are on the basis of a proper understanding of the scientific and clinical evidence and the quality of that evidence, an understanding of the relevant ethical and scientific arguments, an appreciation of the effects of illness on those who are ill, and a lay perspective. In order to further ensure that the decisions taken are reasonable, the group must articulate the reasons for its decisions and make these public. To further the accountability of the decisions an appeals process should be in place.

This process has the following features: decisions are public; the *reasons* for the decisions made are specified; and the decisions made may be appealed against. These features have an important practical implication. The decisions and the reasons for them must, over time, be consistent with each other. If they are not consistent then an appeal can be made along the lines that this decision, or the reasons given for it, are not consistent with a previous decision. In other words, the process has similarities with courts of law: the decisions made in one case at one time cannot be unrelated to relevant decisions made in previous cases.

Three support roles for medical ethics

There are, we believe, three roles for the medical ethicist in supporting resource allocation decisions. The first role involves specifying what a fair procedure will require in making these difficult decisions, and ensuring that this procedure operates appropriately. We call this taking a medical ethics *architect* role. As architect, the ethicist designs the process and its component parts. In practice where this has been done, the procedure normally involves one or more committees. The architect's role will involve specifying a committee's makeup and operating procedures. It might also require clarifying fair processes in the committee's deliberations. For example, NICE takes the view that a fair and accountable decision-making process is one in which an appointed *Citizens Council* can devise and review Social Value

Judgements—those ethical principles that should be reasoned out within the process of the fair allocation of resources.

The second role sees the medical ethicist in her familiar guise as *facilitator*. Similar to the role adopted in Chapter 6, she helps the committee to clarify and articulate its ethical reasoning around each specific decision that it makes, and within the broad framework of fair decision-making that the committee has adopted. By building the structure of reasoning that leads to, and supports, its decisions, the committee is able to demonstrate that it operates consistently and coherently. There is a close relationship between the medical ethicist acting as architect and facilitator. This is because the very act of making decisions helps to develop the relevant principles and shapes how a fair procedure can best operate. Over time, as decisions are taken and the reasons for them are articulated, it becomes possible to gather together the ethical basis on which decisions are made. This guidance can then be fed back into how the committee operates, and into those bodies (such as NICE's Citizens Council) that are convened to give shape to the ethical principles all committees are required to consider.

The third and final role sees the ethicist acting as *judge*. A resource allocation committee is tasked with making a decision about whether or not to fund a particular treatment. If the ethicist is a member of such a committee she is part of the decision-making body and ought to express her substantive ethical views about the right decision to make. In so doing, she is sitting as one of a number of individuals on the committee, and her judgement would count equally with those of her fellow committee members.

In all these supportive roles, reasoning and argument lie at the heart of the contribution that medical ethics makes.

Let us return now to the medical ethicist operating in the third role and consider one of the ethical values with which most healthcare systems have to grapple. This has come to be known as the *rule of rescue*.

The rule of rescue

The rule of rescue is a principle that is relevant when there is a person (or people) whose life is at particularly high risk, but where there is an intervention ('rescue') which has a chance of saving the person's life. The value that is at the heart of the rule of rescue is this: that it is normally justified to spend more, per year of life gained, in a situation where we know, and can *see*, that we have helped a particular person than when we cannot identify who has been helped. For example, that we should be prepared to spend more (perhaps much more) to save the life of a Tony Bullimore than, for example, we would be prepared to spend, *per life saved*, on road safety measures or public health campaigns. In contrast to cost-effectiveness, this principle is guided by the idea that a person is not merely the bearer of good outcomes.

To help understand the rule of rescue in more detail consider two hypothetical (but realistic) situations in Box 11.

According to the rule of rescue it may be right to fund intervention B but not intervention A, even though B is less cost-effective. In practice this is often what happens. If the money spent on some people for renal dialysis were, instead, spent on some people with moderately raised cholesterol, five times as many years of life might be gained. But we don't do it because we would feel that we had condemned identifiable people in high need of dialysis to death; whereas all we would be doing in the case of not funding statins for people with moderately raised cholesterol would be lowering slightly an already quite small chance of death for a large group of (statistical) patients.

A handful of thought experiments can help us to ascertain arguments in favour and against this principle.

Box 11 Comparing two interventions

Intervention A (saves anonymous 'statistical' lives)

A is a drug which will reduce the chance of death by a small amount in a large number of people. For example, out of every 2,000 people in the relevant group, if A is not given then a hundred people will die over the next few years. If A is given then only ninety-eight will die. Although we know that drug A will prevent deaths, we do not know which specific people's lives will be saved. Drug A is cheap—the cost per year of life gained is £20,000. One example of a medical treatment like this are medicines known as statins that lower blood cholesterol. Lowering cholesterol reduces the risk of heart attack, stroke, and death. In this case, if the drug is made available, we know that we have saved lives, but there is no way of identifying the specific people whose lives have been saved.

Intervention B (rescues identified people)

B is the only effective treatment for an otherwise life-threatening condition that affects a relatively small number of people. Those with the condition face a greater than 90 per cent chance of death over the next year if not given B. If given B then there is a good chance of cure—say 90 per cent. B is expensive. The cost per year of life gained is £50,000. Renal (kidney) dialysis is an example of this type. In this case, if dialysis is given to a specific person, we know that we have saved the person's life. If we do not give dialysis, we know that we will not save the person's life.

Two thought experiments that support the rule of rescue

The two of us enjoy cycling around the streets in our home town of Oxford (Figure 8). In doing this we are putting ourselves at only a small extra risk of premature death. In balancing risks and benefits we find that the pleasure of cycling—a really rather

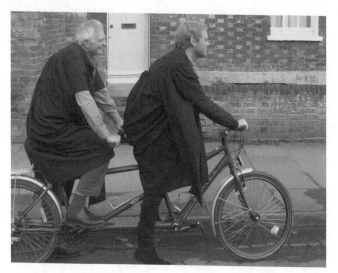

8. Tandem cycling.

small pleasure in both of our lives—outweighs this extra risk.
There seems nothing irrational in this. A very small chance
of a terrible harm is itself only a small negative weight easily
outweighed by other benefits. Most of us will take such small
risks not only for our own benefit but for the benefit of others.

Consider now a friend's job application. Suppose our friend
is applying for a job he is keen to get. To meet the deadline,
the application must be posted today. Owing to a severe bout of
influenza, our friend cannot do this himself. To assist, we cycle
to his house to post the application for him. Again, this action
increases by a very small amount our chance of premature death.
This is easily outweighed by the value of helping our friend.

With these considerations in mind, we propose an argument in
favour of paying for a 'rescue' intervention of type B (at, for example,
a cost of £50,000 per year of life gained) while refusing to pay for
an anonymous 'statistical' intervention of type A (at, for example,

a cost of only £20,000 per year of life gained). We will make the argument using statins as an example of the 'statistical' intervention, and renal dialysis as an example of the rescue intervention.

Those who would benefit from statin treatments gain very little—a very small reduction in the risk of premature death. The 'friend's job application' shows that we readily risk small changes in the risk of premature death, even for benefits to others. Even if we ourselves stood to gain from statins (because we had moderately raised cholesterol levels) it would be reasonable, and not extraordinarily altruistic, for us to prefer that the money goes towards renal dialysis for someone who would otherwise die. From the policy-makers' perspective, it certainly seems better to keep a few people alive (who would otherwise certainly die) than to reduce only slightly the chance of death of many people, particularly when the risk of premature death is fairly low anyway.

One thought experiment against the rule of rescue

We will now discuss a thought experiment that argues against the rule of rescue. Consider the case of a trapped miner (see Box 12), and suppose the facts are these: there is a small risk of death to those in the rescue party, and this risk varies according to the size of the rescue party. If there are a hundred rescuers there would be a 1:1,000 chance of death for each rescuer. If 10,000 rescuers then each would face a 1:5,000 chance of death. If 100,000 rescuers (an extraordinarily large rescue party—but this is a 'thought experiment' to test a theoretical point) then each would face a 1:10,000 risk.

Thus, the larger the rescue party, the smaller the risk of death faced by each individual rescuer. It is also the case, however, that the larger the rescue party, the more people are likely to die in the rescue attempt. With a rescue party of 100,000, each member of

Box 12 The case of the trapped miner

A miner lies trapped following an accident. Without rescue he will die. Given a sufficiently large rescue party the miner can be saved.

Two questions for the reader:

1. Do you think you should join the rescue party if you face a 1:10,000 risk of death in so doing?

2. Is there any further key information you need to know before you can answer the first question?

the rescue party faces a very small risk of death—well within the risks that we normally take for much less important gains than saving a life. However in a rescue party of this size about ten people are expected to die in order to save only one person.

We assume that most people are altruistic at least to a small extent, and most people will accept a very small risk of personal death in order to save another's life. We also assume, further, that most people, given the choice, would like to face as low a personal risk of death as possible. If these assumptions are correct, then respecting the wishes of each potential member of the rescue party would have the following result: an enormous rescue party should be convened, at the expense of many lives. Thus, if the issue of rescue is seen simply as a question of balancing individual risks for each rescuer against the benefit to the individual of being rescued, it would seem right to pursue a policy which overall was very costly in terms of lives lost. We would be embarking on a rescue in which around ten people will die to save one person.

Returning to statins and renal dialysis, it is not clear if those who could benefit from the anonymous 'statistical' intervention have voluntarily agreed to forego their treatment in order for identifiable patients to receive expensive life-extending treatment. Spending more per year of life gained on rescue treatments than on 'statistical' treatments, is effectively volunteering those who would benefit from the preventive treatment to take part in a 'rescue party' for those requiring the rescue treatment. In the absence of a clear mandate from the group of people who stand to lose by a particular decision, we are sceptical about whether it would be right for a healthcare system to let more die to save a few.

But is this conclusion acceptable? Let's go back to Tony Bullimore and the dramatic, successful rescue undertaken by the Australian defence forces. Only a stone-hearted theorist could read Bullimore's account and conclude that it was wrong to mount this rescue. Thus, the defence forces were right to spend millions of taxpayers' money. In the same way, a society should spend £50,000 a year to keep a patient alive on renal dialysis because we cannot stand by and say to that patient: we could keep you alive for many years but we will not do so as we have other priorities. And how could we say this to the relatives who would face bereavement?

The Bullimore case seems very different from the patient with moderately raised cholesterol. Without treatment, the chances are that any individual person will not have a heart attack and die. By refusing the treatment we are not condemning each individual to death as we are doing to the renal patient but instead are only very slightly increasing what remains a small chance of death. But the logic of the trapped miner case gives reason to pause before concluding that renal dialysis should take precedence over statins. It is true that in not providing treatment for the raised cholesterol, we do so not knowing which specific people will die as a result of lack of treatment nor which relatives will then be bereaved. But we do know that there will be such people. Is it not a lack of moral imagination for us to discount death and suffering simply because we cannot know which specific people will have been fatally affected?

Putting principles into practice

Exploring the knotty issue of health resource allocation has shown that medical ethics can play supportive roles in policy-making decisions that go beyond its role in supporting decision-making within patient care settings. The medical ethicist acts as the architect of a process of fair and accountable decision-making, and she also facilitates discussion about, and judges between, those ethical values that have been identified for application within this process. Ultimately, however, it is the quality of the process—not the judgement of the medical ethicist or any other single member of the committee—that determines precisely how these principles should be reasoned through and applied in practice.

In Chapters 4 and 5 we showed medical ethics challenging conventional thinking. In this and the previous chapter we have seen medical ethics supporting decision-making. But is medical ethics always helpful? We now turn to areas where medical ethics is under threat: to two settings in which it is frequently claimed that medical ethics undermines rather than advances good decision-making.

Chapter 8
How modern genetics is testing traditional confidentiality

In Chapters 4 and 5 we saw medical ethics challenging both current clinical practice and the ways in which society treats people with mental illness. In Chapters 6 and 7 we portrayed medical ethics as helper and support. Now we will see medical ethics itself under challenge. One area of challenge comes from developments in medical science and technology—developments that raise new ethical questions or old questions in new ways.

Modern reproductive techniques, for example, can result in biological connections between parents and children that are novel. The woman who contributes half the genetic makeup of the child can now be a different person from the woman who carries the foetus to term. Recent techniques enable more than two people to contribute genetic material to the embryo. It will soon be possible for an embryo to be created from the genetic material of two men; or from two women; or to create embryos from combinations of genetic material from both humans and non-human animals; and perhaps even to create human embryos completely synthetically. An ethics based on concepts such as parental rights, or even human rights, may need to be radically re-interpreted, or re-thought. Technologies that may at first appear to raise major new ethical issues, however, can become routine, with few people continuing to find them ethically problematic or complex. Such has been the case with organ transplants between humans and the use of, for example, pig heart valves in treating human disease. Whether the same will be true in the case of all the modern reproductive technologies remains to be seen.

We don't have to gaze into the future, however, to see medical ethics under challenge from the capabilities of modern technology. The everyday work of genetics clinics all over the world is forcing us to re-think the traditional ways in which we consider medical confidentiality.

Modern genetics, increasingly, enables us both to reveal the past and to foretell the future. And it goes further. A genetic test from one person can provide information about a relative. This was possible to a limited extent before modern genetics. What is new is the extent to which these possibilities can be realized.

Let us start with the revealing of secrets. Box 13 outlines a realistic case from a genetics service.

Box 13 Case 1: genetic tests reveal secrets of paternity

A couple, Robert and Hannah, have a baby who is born with an undiagnosed genetic disorder. Robert and Hannah wish to know the chance that any future child of theirs will be similarly affected. To answer this question the genomes of Robert, Hannah, and the baby are sequenced and compared. This analysis reveals that Robert was not in fact the baby's biological father and that the baby's condition is the result of the unfortunate combination of a sequence in Hannah's genome with that of whoever was the biological father of the baby. The baby's disorder is genetically like that of classical recessive inheritance. This means that the chance of any child of Hannah's having the condition depends on who is the biological father.

If it is the same man as the father of her baby then that chance is 25 per cent (see Figure 9). A future baby who is the biological child of Hannah and Robert, however, is very unlikely to have the disorder. This is because Robert has two copies of the normal gene that will prevent his children from having the disorder.

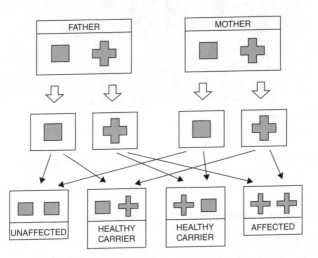

9. **Autosomal recessive inheritance.**

Should the geneticist disclose, to Robert, the finding that he is not the father of the baby (see Figure 10)? Guidelines for practitioners vary in the advice they give on this.

Many geneticists would be prepared to tell a lie or fudge the issue, for example by claiming that the child with the condition has the condition as a result of a new mutation, rather than being honest with their patient. A survey of patients, as opposed to doctors, carried out in the US suggested that three-quarters thought that the doctor ought to tell the husband that he is not

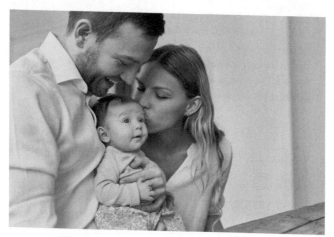

10. **Couple with baby.**

the father of the child, at least if he asks directly. The majority of those in that survey were women.

Medical confidentiality

Hippocrates was born on the Greek island of Cos in about 460 BC. The Hippocratic Oath is one of the earliest known sets of professional guidelines for doctors. Some of the guidelines now seem dated but what the Oath says about confidentiality is still relevant: 'Whatever I may see or learn about people in the course of my work or in my private life which should not be disclosed I will keep to myself and treat in complete confidence'.

In order to pursue the question of the limits of confidentiality compare Case 1 with Case 2 (in Box 14, presented and drawn from a paper published in *The Lancet* by Parker and Lucassen).

In Case 2, it would be widely accepted that the doctor should not breach the confidentiality of Mary.

Box 14 Case 2: paternity revealed by the mother

'following a healthy pregnancy and birth Mary visits her general practitioner for her routine 6-week postnatal visit. Mary's husband, Peter, is registered with the same GP. During the consultation Mary reveals that Peter is not the father of her child' (see Notes and references).

The guidelines provided by the General Medical Council (GMC), the professional body for UK doctors, state that disclosure of personal information without consent may be justified when there is a public interest in doing so. For the GMC, this public interest arises when the disclosure of personal information is necessary to protect other individuals in society from 'a risk of death or serious harm'.

In applying guidelines to a particular situation some interpretation is needed. In this case such interpretation seems relatively straightforward. The harm of not telling Peter does not amount to 'a risk of death or serious harm'. The doctor, therefore, should not breach Mary's confidentiality.

Comparing Cases 1 and 2

If the doctor should not breach confidentiality in Case 2, does it follow that the geneticist should keep quiet about the question of paternity in Case 1?

There are important differences between the two cases. In Case 1, the fact of non-paternity was discovered as a result of tests for which both Robert and Hannah gave consent. In Case 2 this fact was revealed only by Mary. In Case 1, Robert and Hannah came to the geneticist together to discuss an issue of joint concern. The information concerning paternity is directly relevant to the issue about which Robert and Hannah came jointly to see the geneticist.

The foundations of medical confidentiality

The case comparison may leave us in doubt about what the geneticist should do in Case 1. Consideration of Case 2 provides some reasons why the geneticist should keep information about paternity secret from Robert. But Case 2 differs from Case 1 in some important respects that might make all the difference.

Perhaps we can be helped by going back to theory and asking the question: what are the fundamental reasons why maintaining medical confidentiality is important. The three most commonly given answers to this question are: respect for patient autonomy; to keep an implied promise; and to bring about the best consequences.

Foundation 1: respect for patient autonomy

The principle of respect for patient autonomy (see Chapter 3) emphasizes the patient's right to have control over her own life. It implies that a person has the right, by and large, to decide who should have access to information about himself (i.e. a right to privacy). On this view the patient who reveals information about herself to the doctor has the right to determine who else, if anyone, should know that information. The doctor should not normally pass that information on to a third party without the patient's permission.

Foundation 2: implied promise

Some argue that the relationship between doctor and patient includes implied understandings, one of which is that the doctor will not breach patient confidentiality. On this view the reason why a doctor should not breach confidentiality is because to do so would involve breaching an understanding which amounts to breaking a promise.

Foundation 3: best consequences

A major group of theories in moral philosophy (consequentialism) claims that the right action in any situation is the one that will have the best (foreseeable) consequences. On this view, the reasons why doctors should maintain confidentiality would be because so doing leads to the best consequences. Only if doctors are strict in maintaining confidentiality will patients trust them. And such trust is vital if patients are to seek and obtain the necessary help from doctors.

Do these theories help us in answering the question: should the geneticist tell Robert that he is not the father of the newborn baby?

The theory of respect for autonomy is ambiguous when we try to apply it to Case 1. It all depends on a decision regarding on whose autonomy we focus. Robert's autonomy is respected by telling Robert; Hannah's by keeping it secret from Robert (unless Hannah gives permission to tell Robert).

The implied promise theory is similarly problematic. In normal clinical practice as exemplified by Case 2, it is clear that the patient (Mary) can expect the doctor to respect her confidentiality. But it is not so clear what the implied promise is in Case 1. This theory, however, suggests a practical way forward in future cases: that it should be made clear to patients before any testing is carried out what approach to information-sharing the clinic will take.

A consequentialist account certainly gives reasons why the doctor in Case 1 should keep the paternity issue secret from Robert on grounds of the possible deleterious effect on the family. This is the main reason why many geneticists would not tell Robert that he is not the biological father of Hannah's child. But it is not clear that the consequences of keeping Robert ignorant are better than informing him of the truth. Is it right that Hannah needs to be protected from the consequences of her behaviour and will it be better for the family if it remains a secret? This is an example of a major practical problem with consequentialism: it is often impossible to determine with sufficient degree of certainty what the various consequences of different courses of action are likely to be.

Examining the theories of what underpins the moral importance of confidentiality appears to have been of no more help than case comparison. The difficulty, we believe, is that we have been focusing on the wrong aspect of the problem. The key question is not whether there are sufficient grounds, in terms of Robert's interests, for breaching Hannah's confidentiality. The question is whether the information that the newborn baby is not Robert's biological baby, is as much 'his information' as Hannah's. Whose information is it? Let us examine this question through the lens of a third case, presented in Box 15, and drawn from a paper published by Parker and Lucassen in the *British Medical Journal*:

Box 15 Case 3: secrets and sisters

A 4-year-old boy was diagnosed with Duchenne muscular dystrophy (DMD). DMD is a severe, debilitating, and progressive muscle-wasting disease in which children become wheelchair-bound by their early teens and often die in their 20s. It is an X-linked recessive condition and so only boys are affected. The boy's mother, Helen, was found to be a carrier for the mutation. Women who are carriers do not show symptoms of the condition, but half of their sons will inherit it from them and will be affected.

Helen had a sister, Penelope, who was ten weeks' pregnant. Penelope's obstetrician referred her to the genetics team after she told him that her nephew had speech and development delay. She told him that although she was not close to her sister and had not discussed it with her, she was concerned about the implications for her own pregnancy. Penelope made it clear that she would consider terminating a pregnancy if she knew that the foetus was affected with a serious inherited condition. Speech and development delay are features of a range of conditions and would not of themselves have indicated carrier-testing for DMD. Because there are a number of possible mutations of the DMD gene, testing without information about which mutation was responsible for the nephew's condition would have been unlikely to be informative.

At the next meeting with her clinical geneticist, Helen says that she knows that her sister is pregnant and that she understands that the pregnancy could be affected. She also says that she has not discussed this with her sister, partly because they don't really get on, but also because she suspects that if her sister were to find out, and if the foetus turned out to be affected, she would terminate the pregnancy. Helen feels very strongly that this would be wrong. She knows that her sister does not share her views, but Helen says that she has decided that she wants her test results and information about her son to remain confidential (see Notes and references).

We want to put aside the question of whether Penelope should or should not have a termination if her foetus carries the gene and focus on the issue of confidentiality. Parker and Lucassen propose two models of confidentiality: the personal account model and the joint account model (see Notes and references).

The personal account model

The personal account model is the conventional view of medical confidentiality. On this view the information about Helen's genetic state—as a carrier of Duchenne's muscular dystrophy (DMD)—'belongs' to Helen, and Helen alone. Respect for such confidentiality is important. It has, however, long been recognized that there are limits to such confidentiality, as has already been highlighted by the GMC criteria quoted earlier. But these limits are the exception. On this view the key question is whether the foreseeable harms to Penelope if the information is not disclosed are sufficiently serious to justify breaching Helen's confidentiality.

The joint account model

On the joint account model, genetic information, like information about a joint bank account, is shared by more than one person. Helen's request, on this view, would be analogous to asking the bank manager not to reveal information about a joint account to the other account-holders. On this view genetic information should be seen in a completely different way from most medical information when that information identifies a familial factor. It is information that should be available to all 'account holders'—in other words, to all (close) genetically related family members. That is, unless there are good reasons to withhold the information.

These two models see the onus of proof, with respect to sharing information, in opposite ways. On the conventional, personal account, model we ask: are the harms to Penelope so great that they override Helen's right to confidentiality? On the joint account model the genetic information, although obtained from Helen's blood and medical history, 'belongs' to the family and should be made available for the care of all family members. Penelope has a right to information about the familial factor as it is key information to help her to know important aspects of her genetic makeup that could improve her health outcomes. There would need to be very good reasons, in terms of Helen's interests, to justify denying Penelope access to the genetic test for DMD. Penelope's right to genetic information is limited, however. Her claim to access information about the familial genetic factor does not mean that she has any right to information about Helen's health condition or medical care.

Helen knows something not only about herself and her son but also about Penelope and *her* unborn child. Helen knows that Penelope's foetus has a significant chance of suffering from DMD, but Penelope does not know this. This asymmetry of knowledge is unfair to Penelope. The personal account model fails to take this fact into account.

We suggest that modern genetics has forced us to re-consider the status of some medical information. By applying medical ethicists' well-honed tools of reasoning and argument we have suggested that the conventional view that genetic information should be regarded as private to an individual is unsound. Our analysis aims to show that the guidelines developed by the profession on the basis of medical ethical analysis need to be re-considered and amended in light of new arguments. It is important that guidelines (and broader regulatory frameworks such as national laws) are not set in stone, and that these adapt as arguments evolve in the face of technological advances in healthcare. Our view is that the GMC should embrace and incorporate the joint account model in order to guide how genetic information is handled appropriately within families and to consider it as belonging, potentially, to a group of people and not to the individual patient. The traditional individualistic model of patient confidentiality may need to adapt.

In the next chapter we will again question the overarching trend in contemporary medical ethics to take an individualistic approach to clarifying ethical values and duties. It is not only advances in science and technology that require us to re-consider our long-standing ethical positions. Cultural differences within and across societies can also challenge our assumptions and approaches to medical ethics. As with new technologies, cultural differences require us to re-consider our ethical obligations to individuals, and to pay close attention to the ways in which relationships within communities vary across different societies. Medical research involving collaboration between widely varying cultures is one context which is particularly problematic. It is to this topic that we now turn.

Chapter 9
Culture, consent, and community

Tomorrow's medicine is today's research. That is why the question of how we prioritize and carry out medical research is at least as important as the question of how we prioritize and practice healthcare itself. Medical research is in many ways more strictly regulated than medical practice. From a perusal of the innumerable guidelines on medical research you could be forgiven for thinking that medical research, like smoking, must be bad for your health; that in a liberal society, since it cannot be altogether banned, strict regulation is needed to minimize the harm that it can do.

The reason for this strict control lies in history. L.P. Hartley begins his novel *The Go-Between* with the sentence 'The past is a foreign country: they do things differently there.' It was the appalling experiments carried out by some Nazi doctors that led, in 1946, to the first internationally agreed guidelines on medical research involving people—the Nuremberg Code.

It was not only in Nazi Germany, however, that people were grossly abused in the interests of medical research. A study of syphilis undertaken in the 1970s by the US Public Health Service in Tuskegee in the US deliberately left untreated over 400 poor black men who were suffering from syphilis in order to research the natural course of the disease. The men were recruited under the guise of free healthcare, but were denied the penicillin treatment that could have ameliorated their symptoms.

The Nuremberg Code led to the Declaration of Helsinki which was first published by the World Medical Association in 1964 and last updated in 2013. This Declaration has many offspring, of varying legitimacy, in the form of guidelines for medical research. The guidelines highlight four main ethical issues: respect for the autonomy of the potential participants in research; protection of participants from the risk of harm; the value and quality of the research; and aspects of justice. In addition, research ethics committees have been created to scrutinize planned medical research to ensure that the ethical guidelines are followed.

Governing research: three criticisms

Although the ethical principles that inform the regulation of medical research include valuing the good, for people in the future, that can come from the research, the main focus of the guidelines and of the process of regulation has been the research participants: their autonomy and protection. This has led to criticism, especially from researchers and advocates of evidence-based medicine, of current regulation and processes, and of the part played by medical ethicists. There are three principal criticisms.

First, that the regulation process significantly delays research, leading to delays in reaping the benefits of the research and to lives being lost.

Second, that guidelines are too paternalistic towards participants. Most guidelines state that research participants should not be put at more than 'minimal risk of harm'. This is the case even if the participant is a competent adult fully informed about the risks and benefits and who voluntarily agrees to take part. Although it is not entirely clear what is meant by minimal harm, it seems to be set at a level taken by somewhat risk-averse people in their normal lives. Critics of the guidelines ask why risk of harm should be more carefully controlled and more restrictive, in the context of medical research, than it is in other areas of our lives. We do not prevent the sale or purchase of skis, motorbikes, or hang-gliders, although these expose purchasers to moderate risks. Why should the control of medical research be different?

Third, that the amount of information provided to participants who are being asked to take part in medical research is substantial and much greater than the level of information that would be normal in clinical practice. Critics claim that this is an example of 'double standards'—an indefensible difference in information level between the research and the clinical settings. Double standards are an example of inconsistency.

Disagreements between the advocates and the critics of current guidelines and regulation may be hard to resolve. There may be differences of view about the relative weights to be given to respect for autonomy on the one hand, and the good from the research, to people in the future, on the other hand. There may in addition be disagreements over whether the same level of information should be provided in the contexts of clinical care and medical research. The arguments on both sides, however, will share a common ethical framework and a common understanding of the values at stake. The criticisms do not undermine the discipline of medical ethics as we have presented it in this book. Quite the contrary, the criticisms are themselves examples of the practice of the discipline.

Governing international research: Western imperialism?

This is not clearly the case, however, with another kind of attack on the ethical regulation of medical research. The core of this attack is the claim that the ethical regulation of medical research is a modern example of *imperialism*—of Western countries imposing their views and practices on non-Western countries, that have quite different cultures (see Notes and references).

Many diseases affect those in non-Western countries to a much greater extent than those in Western countries. Malaria is an example. Non-Western countries that have low gross domestic products (GDPs) per capita cannot typically afford much medical research. It is quite proper therefore for institutions in Western countries to fund, and use their facilities to support, medical research in non-Western countries—research that will involve participants in those countries and that is likely to lead to health benefits for those populations.

Medical research is becoming increasingly international in scope. For pharmaceutical companies, exporting their research activities into non-Western countries has helped to cut the costs of conducting large-scale medical trials, and may also bring research activity closer to new markets for the products being tested. For academic institutions, global health research has gained prominence because of the increasing recognition of the huge mortality and morbidity that results from untreated diseases in non-Western countries. Large-scale research studies into these diseases are typically run in partnership between Western universities and research institutions newly established in non-Western countries.

With the lessons from the syphilis study at Tuskegee in mind it will be important not to exploit the participants in research carried out in non-Western countries. Those lessons suggest that research in non-Western countries should be regulated in the same way, using the same ethical principles, as research in Western countries. It is no surprise therefore that the Council for International Organizations of Medical Sciences laid down the following position in the preamble to its 2016 guidelines: 'The ethical principles set forth in these Guidelines should be upheld in the ethical review of research protocols. The ethical principles are regarded as universal.' Marcia Angell, a former editor of a leading medical journal—*The New England Journal of Medicine*—wrote: 'Human subjects in any part of the world should be protected by an irreducible set of ethical standards.'

Individual informed consent is the main approach to protecting the rights and welfare of research participants in Western countries. Valid consent requires the person to be provided with relevant information, to have the ability to make an informed choice, and to be free from undue influence or coercion such that the person is making his own free choice. Consent in the setting of research in Western countries is typically standardized by a research team using an information sheet, the contents of which depend on the nature of the research procedures. A consent form is usually signed by each individual participant to convey her agreement. Figure 11 provides an example of such a consent form.

In order, therefore, not to exploit research participants in non-Western countries, the research frameworks and codes of ethics developed in Europe and North America, and supported by the major Western funders, have been used to regulate research in poor countries. Research ethics committees have been established in the local hospitals that host research, and the very same considerations of participants' welfare and rights used in Western countries are expected to be given due attention by those researchers working across national borders.

Although exporting these Western notions of valid consent (and the other ethical principles) to non-Western countries might sound like a decent approach to prevent exploitation of research participants in these countries, is it not yet another example of Western imperialism?

(Form to be on headed paper)

IRAS ID:

Centre Number:

Study Number:

Participant Identification Number for this trial:

CONSENT FORM

Title of Project:

Name of Researcher:

Please initial box

1. I confirm that I have read the information sheet dated.................. (version............) for the above study. I have had the opportunity to consider the information, ask questions and have had these answered satisfactorily.

2. I understand that my participation is voluntary and that I am free to withdraw at any time without giving any reason, without my medical care or legal rights being affected.

3. (If appropriate) I understand that relevant sections of my medical notes and data collected during the study, may be looked at by individuals from [company name], from regulatory authorities or from the NHS Trust, where it is relevant to my taking part in this research. I give permission for these individuals to have access to my records.

4. (If appropriate) I understand that the information collected about me will be used to support other research in the future, and may be shared anonymously with other researchers.

5. (If appropriate) I agree to my General Practitioner being informed of my participation in the study. / I agree to my General Practitioner being involved in the study, including any necessary exchange of information about me between my GP and the research team.

6. (If appropriate) I understand that the information held and maintained by the Health and Social Care Information Centre (or amend as appropriate) and other central UK NHS bodies may be used to help contact me or provide information about my health status.

7. I agree to take part in the above study.

_____   _____   _____
Name of Participant   Date   Signature

_____   _____   _____
Name of Person   Date   Signature
taking consent

When completed: 1 for participant; 1 for researcher site file; 1 to be kept in medical notes.

11. Research consent form.

Consent under challenge

Some people have argued that people living in locations such as rural Kenya, where, for example, important malaria research is being carried out, do not always make decisions, including decisions about whether to participate in research, as individuals carving out their own unique and independent paths through life based on their personal interests and values. Decisions might be made in more complex ways that involve village elders, heads of families, and other processes that reflect the person's membership of a local tribe or village group. Or, they might be deferred entirely to another person—perhaps to an elder member of that community, or, in the case of women, to the husband or head of household within a family setting. Imposing the value of respecting individual autonomy, which gives shape to the requirement to obtain individual valid consent, so the argument goes, is to impose the Western value of extreme individualism—a value that has resulted from the West's history and culture, and a value that may be less dominant in Kenyan culture.

One way to avoid such imposition of values would be for researchers from Western countries and institutions to avoid carrying out any research in non-Western countries. The consequence would be that, for a long time to come, there would be little or no medical research that could effectively help reduce the morbidity and mortality from many of the diseases that cause so much suffering in non-Western countries with lower GDPs per capita. This would seem a total abdication of the responsibility that richer nations have to help poorer nations and therefore unethical.

A more reasonable response would be for researchers from Western countries working in non-Western countries to accept whatever the norms are for consent in the culture in which the research is taking place. In some cultures, this might mean abandoning individual consent entirely. Instead, permission for a person to be recruited into research, or for a blood sample to be taken as part of the research, might be required from a community leader, or from another member of the person's household.

Abandoning the requirement for individual consent entirely is, however, problematic. Adherence to local norms might actively go against the interests of the individual participant, or her values. Even though it may be commonly the case in that person's daily life that decisions are made by others—her husband or an elder perhaps—the commitment to consent in research ethics is born out of a requirement to show a fundamental respect to the individual as a person who is capable of making decisions. A complete adherence to local norms might require the Western researchers to act in ways, and to give support to practices, that they consider ethically wrong. As Kamuya and colleagues consider in relation to taking blood samples, this might mean proceeding with the consent only from the husband, or the village elder, and without enabling the woman herself to refuse.

There is a third response that requires the ethicist to get up from the philosopher's proverbial armchair. To meet the challenge of conflicts of cultures requires more from Western medical ethics than careful thought, analysis, and argument. It requires *engagement*: systematic dialogue, discussion, and involvement with the other culture, which may itself be culturally diverse. This response neither seeks to build local consensus around the force of universal ethical principles nor does it require these principles to be set aside to embrace local social and cultural norms. The way forward, it seems to us, in developing ethically robust research involving researchers and participants from widely differing cultures might be described as *respectful collaboration*. Let's see how this might work in practice.

Respectful collaboration in practice

A practical starting point for the kind of respectful collaboration that we endorse is to establish community advisory boards (CABs), as has been done in HIV research studies undertaken in Cambodia and Nigeria. These boards are a gathering of people within a community who share a common identity, history, language, and culture, but bearing in mind that the communities in which the research is undertaken may be culturally diverse. Convening a CAB requires obtaining authentic community representation, and for the power dynamics between the relevant community members to be replicated. Sometimes the CAB's makeup will reflect a group of village elders who typically take responsibility for matters affecting the community. At other times the CAB might be made up of a wider range of local people who share responsibility among themselves for resolving issues that attain to the community as a whole (see Figure 12). Community

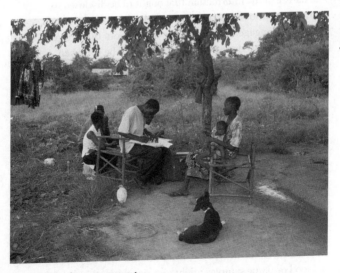

12. Community engagement.

engagement aims to address the challenge to Western notions
of consent in three main ways.

Aim 1: tailoring and disseminating knowledge about how consent processes should operate

The first aim of community engagement is to ensure that informed
consent, and the procedures for obtaining consent, are appropriate
for the local population from whom research participants will be
drawn. This local population will often have limited understanding
of healthcare, research, or the social requirements of giving
consent. A CAB may make it clear that the Western approach
for obtaining written and signed consent is inappropriate.
A more informal approach to working with a participant over
time, and without the use of written documents, may be more
in keeping with local practices and better understood by
potential participants.

The nature of the information that ought to be disclosed to
participants prior to recruitment can also be shaped through
community engagement. Extensive detail about the nature of
the medical procedures involved will need to be conveyed
straightforwardly, making use of local languages perhaps, or the
pictorial display of information. Some information that would
otherwise not be covered in a standard consent process might need
to be disclosed. For example, medical research will often require
taking blood or other biological samples. The analysis of these
samples may be best carried out in rich countries which have better
equipped laboratories than in the non-Western country from
where the samples have been taken. Ethics research undertaken by
Paulina Tindana and colleagues in Ghana, however, has shown
that the local significance attached to blood products can mean
that taking the blood and tissue samples to another country for
analysis gives rise to specific concerns for local participants.
In some cases, the degree of concern that is raised by the exporting
of blood or tissue samples might give rise to an ethical claim to

establish local equipment for sample analysis, rather than simply by making modifications to the consent process.

CABs established in Kenya have shown that researchers may need to adopt an educational role alongside the process of obtaining consent. The employees at a local medical research institution that has been built to carry out the research may also be involved in providing healthcare. Potential participants in the research may have limited understanding of these two distinct roles: carrying out research, and providing healthcare. Any consent process is likely to have to explain basic facts about healthcare, treatment, and the relationship between treatment and research.

Aim 2: clarifying and establishing appropriate routes for recruitment

The second aim of community engagement is to modify standard methods for contacting and recruiting participants. One important development has been for fieldworkers to play a major recruiting role. These fieldworkers are members of the local community employed to carry out the research procedures involved in the studies, taking samples and collecting other kinds of research data. It is they, rather than researchers from the Western institutions, who initiate contact with local people and take the lead in obtaining consent. CABs help to make decisions about where these fieldworkers should obtain permission, often necessitating visits to people's private homes.

Guidance from CABs is likely to play a crucial role in helping researchers to navigate complex local expectations around decision-making and the consent process. For example, if local practice requires women to seek advice about, or to pass over responsibility for, decision-making about health matters to her husband or other male family member, the process through which the woman gives permission should be sensitive to these expectations. Typically, the fieldworker would need to put in place a shared decision-making process. This gives the woman involved overall control over decision-making, but it is also a process in which other people who are typically involved in decision-making in that person's life are encouraged to participate, as long as the woman agrees. For example, a husband can express his views about his wife's participating in the research, and she is able to take these views into account in making a decision about participation. The fieldworker's responsibility is to encourage the woman to consider the different views expressed, alongside her own values, and to make a decision. It is entirely feasible that she will choose to participate because she values the perspective offered by her husband. So long as she has reflected on her decision in this way, this approach shows appropriate respect for her culture, while also respecting the fact that, if she agrees, it is she who will be the subject of the research procedures.

Aim 3: respecting individuals and the communities in which they live

The final aim reflects a more intrinsic feature of community engagement. Creating a CAB can itself help to meet the fundamental requirement to respect individuals. In addition to providing specific guidance about modifying consent, the CAB may adopt a gatekeeping function, determining whether a particular research study is appropriate for local people to participate in at all. Respecting the views and opinions in this way from representatives of the community provides a local body with sufficient power to shape the direction of research practices in light of the values of local people. It is important that the CAB is constructive—that it is generally positive about research—while being also independent of the Western funders and researchers and able to say when the research proposed is inappropriate.

Developing arguments in context

As a product of community engagement, the practice of consent is likely to look very different from standard approaches adopted in medical research carried out in the West. Respecting local people will not give rise to a one-size-fits all standardized consent process. This does not mean that ethical principles underpinning consent and other research requirements are simply discarded to embrace local values. The guiding requirement to respect participants and enable them to have overall control about whether to participate in research is maintained, and will in some cases constrain the degree of adaptation that is made to meet local cultural values and practices.

Progress will depend fundamentally on developing compelling ethical arguments in context, with established rules of argumentation being agreed upon, and shaping the format of discussions between researchers and CABs. Relevant facts about local people's values, beliefs, and expectations should not be set aside by researchers in this process without good reason. Nor can members of the group discard considerations that have overriding ethical force in that context. This includes the value of respecting a person's autonomy, and will also include other values that underpin international research ethics codes: the requirement to obtain a reasonable risk-benefit ratio for participants, and the requirement to treat participants fairly. But progress also depends on the relationships between people. Unless trust and respect is mutual between the various people involved then, however good the arguments, collaborative research will not be possible.

The fundamental methods of medical ethics survive, we believe, the challenges both from developing technology and from the collaborations, and clashes, of cultures. The content, however, the values at stake, and the ways in which these values are balanced, must be kept continually under scrutiny. The future, as well as the past, is indeed a foreign country.

Chapter 10
A glance into the future

The year is 399 BC. Socrates is in court in Athens accused, among other things, of corrupting the youth. He is found guilty.
His accuser proposes one punishment; Socrates has the right to propose an alternative. The court must choose between them.

Socrates begins his speech:

> And so [my accuser] proposes death as the penalty. And what shall
> I propose on my part...?...[I] sought to persuade every man
> among you that he must...seek virtue and wisdom before he looks
> to his private interest.

Socrates considers that he deserves free food provided by the City but realizes that this is unlikely to be the punishment favoured by the court. He ends, more sensibly, by offering to pay a fine, but before he does so he raises the possibility of the one sentence that the court might well have chosen in preference to death.

> And if I say exile...I must indeed be blinded by the love of life,
> if I am so irrational as to expect that when you, who are my own
> citizens, cannot endure my discourses and arguments, and have
> found them so grievous and odious that you will have no more of
> them, others are likely to endure them.

He then considers (but rejects) the possibility of going into exile but ceasing his search, through discussion and debate, for virtue. It is at this point that he makes one of his most famous statements, often translated as: *the unexamined life is not worth living*.

Medical ethics is about the *examined* life, within the broad context of healthcare. As we have seen, this context is relevant to us all. Some work, or are planning to work, as doctors, nurses, or other health professionals. Some work in the community as carers of people disabled in some way by disease. Some of us are thrust into the caring role when illness strikes a relative or friend. Almost all of us become, at times, sick ourselves. And all of us are citizens in a society faced with issues that involve medical ethics: how health resources should be spent; how the seriously mentally ill should be treated both for their own good, and sometimes for the protection of others; what should the limits be, if any, to assisting reproduction or to easing death.

Medical ethics is a practical subject. It is concerned with what is the right thing to do in a particular situation, and often for a particular person. The world is not static and new situations are continually arising. Ethical reasoning, we hope we have demonstrated, is not the application of an algorithm to a situation. It involves the imagination. It involves comparing and contrasting various states of affairs. It makes use of many kinds of argument.

The future of medical ethics, the ways in which it will develop and change, will be largely determined by the nature of the new situations that arise, and we think that these are likely to be of two broad types: scientific and technological developments on the one hand, and social and cultural changes on the other hand.

Scientific and technological developments

The time may not be far off when methods based on genetic and pharmacological advances can be used, not only to prevent disease and disability, but to enhance human beings—for example, to increase intelligence or a person's capacity to act morally. Most of us believe it is right to enhance children's intellectual abilities and moral behaviour through good education, but would it be right to do so through gene therapy, and, if so, under what conditions and with what legal regulation.

Stem cell research has the potential, which is being rapidly realized, of developing novel and effective treatments. Isolated human organs, for example kidneys, and perhaps brains, might be created from a person's cells (e.g. from a person's cheek cells) without creating a human being. Such organs could be immensely valuable in organ transplantation.

Stem cell research will also soon make possible the creation of human beings from two parents of the same sex, or even from the cells of one 'parent'. It is also likely to become possible to create novel creatures that combine human and animal parts.

Synthetic biology, which uses the methods of engineering with biologically active components such as synthetic DNA, could lead to the production of living organisms from non-living components and from DNA sequences never found in nature.

Advances in information technology and artificial intelligence (AI) will lead to increasing use of computers and robots in medical diagnosis and in the delivery of healthcare. With the development of programs that learn and develop independently of human control, and that make medical decisions that cannot be subject to human scrutiny, new and complex issues of accountability and responsibility will arise.

The ability of powerful computers to manage and analyse huge sets of data ('big data') is already leading to difficult issues around consent, confidentiality, and ownership. Health systems are beginning the ambitious goal of improving health outcomes by collecting, storing, and integrating data about patients' genetic makeup, their medical histories, and their broader socio-economic circumstances. But, it is far from clear how patients' consent should be obtained when very little can be known about the intended future use of these datasets, or even whether these patients would have any claim over their data once it has been analysed, adapted, integrated with other patients' data, and analysed further.

Cultural changes and the international context

Medical ethics has been a part of the significant cultural changes that have occurred in many Western countries over recent decades and that have emphasized individual rights and the importance of respect for the autonomy of patients. There seems no reason to suppose that cultural change will now stagnate. Indeed it is likely that change will become increasingly rapid. We saw in Chapter 9 that the international context in which much modern medical research takes place has led to challenges to the primacy and universality of the codes of ethics as they have developed in Western countries. It seems inevitable that over the next decades the international context will become increasingly significant in most areas of our lives, including those relevant to healthcare. This is likely to lead, in all countries, to significant changes, relevant to ethics, as cultures with widely differing religious, social, and family values and practices attempt to cooperate in areas of mutual benefit.

Social media are also having an impact on how medical ethics is developing in different societies and across different cultures. The ability to access and share information enables people, including those in less well-developed countries, to be usefully informed and gives them more power in many situations including in accessing and benefitting from healthcare. Medical ethics itself will become more public with a much wider range of people able to express their views in ways accessible to anyone in the world. These developments might enrich the debates but, at the same time, these media provide a powerful forum for the promulgation of falsehoods, potentially undermining appropriate expertise and sidelining rational argument.

Despite the differences, however, between the present, the past, and what is to come, we believe that the fundamental methods of medical ethics survive. The values at stake and the ways in which these values are balanced must be kept under scrutiny, and will change. But at the core of medical ethics, for it to be medical ethics at all, is the role of reasoning: providing reasons; maintaining consistency across reasons; and being continually open to rational criticism. The challenges from both technology and globalization make it crucially important for medical ethics to continue to progress through the process of rational argument and the assessment of evidence—a process that has developed over the centuries since Socrates walked the streets of Athens, making himself unpopular through questioning the beliefs of his fellow citizens.

Notes and references

Chapter 1: On why medical ethics is exciting

The observation about the Old Masters comes from W.H. Auden's poem *Musée des Beaux Arts*. London: Faber and Faber, 1979.

I. Berlin 1953. *The Hedgehog and the Fox*. London: Weidenfeld and Nicolson.

Z. Smith 2003. Review. *The Guardian* (London), 1 November, p. 6.

Chapter 2: Assisted dying: good medical practice, or murder?

C. Spencer 1996. *Heretic's Feast: A history of vegetarianism*. Dartmouth: University Press of New England.

N. Warburton 2007. *Thinking from A to Z*, 3rd edn. Abingdon: Routledge.

Chapter 3: A toolbox of reasoning

A. Flew 1989. *An Introduction to Western Philosophy*. London: Thames and Hudson.

R. Gillon 1986. *Philosophical Medical Ethics*. Oxford: Wiley & Sons.

R. Nozick 1974. *Anarchy, State, and Utopia*. New York: Basic Books.

N. Warburton 2007. *Thinking from A to Z*, 3rd edn. Abingdon: Routledge.

Chapter 4: People who don't exist; at least not yet

L. Sterne 1760. *The Life and Opinions of Tristram Shandy, Gentleman*. London: Everyman Library, ch. 1.

I. Kennedy and A. Grubb 2000. *Medical Law*, 3rd edn. London: Butterworths, pp. 1272–3.

D. Parfit 1984. *Reasons and Persons*. Oxford: Oxford University Press.

Chapter 5: Inconsistencies about madness

The discussion on protecting society from dangerous people owes a great deal to Harriet Mather who developed many of these ideas in the course of her studies as a medical student.

Chapter 6: Helping the helper

D. Parfit 1984. *Reasons and Persons*. Oxford: Oxford University Press, p. 281.

Chapter 7: Establishing fair procedure

T. Bullimore 1997. *Saved*. London: Time Warner Books. Calculating the cost is not at all straightforward, as Bullimore himself discusses (see p. 293). One could put a price on all the person-hours, the airplane, and the ship usage. This would probably come to several million pounds. Alternatively, you might argue that all the personnel would have been paid anyway—so the only extra cost was the wear and tear on the planes and ships. Or you could say that the rescue was useful training and cost-free. In many situations the cost estimations of healthcare interventions are similarly open to enormous variation depending on what is included in the calculation.

Chapter 8: How modern genetics is testing traditional confidentiality

General Medical Council. 2017. *Confidentiality: Good Practice in Handling Patient Information*. London: GMC. https://www.gmc-uk.org

M. Parker and A. Lucassen 2001. Revealing false paternity: some ethical considerations. *The Lancet*, 357: 1033–5.

M. Parker and A. Lucassen 2004. Genetic information: a joint account? *BMJ*, 329: 165. See also: M. Parker and A. Lucassen 2018. Using a genetic test result in the care of family members: how does the duty of confidentiality apply? *European Journal of Human Genetics*. https://doi.org/10.1038/s41431-018-0138-y

Chapter 9: Culture, consent, and community

We use the terms 'Western' and 'non-Western' countries to differentiate between those parts of the world where international health research is funded and where it is hosted. In relation to the context of claims about imperialism, we think that these two terms are preferable to the following alternatives: 'high income' and 'low income' countries, 'more economically developed' and 'less economically developed' countries, and 'global north' and 'global south'. Hans Rosling, for good reasons, advocates using four levels of income (level 1 being the poorest) in summarizing world data. Kenya and Ghana (the principal 'host' countries in the examples used in this chapter) are classified as level 2, and the US and UK (principal 'funding' countries in the examples used) are classified as level 4 (see https://www.gapminder.org).

D.M. Kamuya, S.J. Theobald, V. Marsh, M. Parker, W.P. Geissler, and S.C. Molyneux. 2015. '*The one who chases you away does not tell you go*': silent refusals and complex power relations in research consent processes in coastal Kenya. *PLoS One*, 10(5): e0126671.

P. Tindana, C.S. Molyneux, S. Bull, and M. Parker. 2014. Ethical issues in the export, storage and reuse of human biological samples in biomedical research: perspectives of key stakeholders in Ghana and Kenya. *BMC Medical Ethics*, 15: 76.

Chapter 10: A glance into the future

The translations of Plato are from *The Apology*, translated by Benjamin Jowett.

Further reading

We hope that this 'taster' of medical ethics has whetted your appetite for the subject. We provide further reading for specific topics, related to each chapter as follows.

Chapter 1: On why medical ethics is exciting

The methods of medical ethics are of course those of ethics more generally; it is the subject matter that is specific. But, having said that, medical ethics is one area of practical ethics that has been particularly innovative in its methodologies. A developing area is the use of empirical methods borrowed from the social sciences. Empirical research and philosophical analysis can be integrated to enrich the quality of arguments in medical ethics. Two good books that discuss the use of different methodolgies and methods are:

J. Sugarman and D. Sulmasy (eds) 2010. *Methods in Medical Ethics*, 2nd edn. Georgetown: Georgetown University Press.

J. Ives, M. Dunn, and A. Cribb (eds) 2016. *Empirical Bioethics: Theoretical and Practical Perspectives*. Cambridge: Cambridge University Press.

There are several encyclopaedias of ethics that provide good introductions to particular topics with useful reference lists. Examples are:

R.F. Chadwick (ed.) 2011. *Encyclopedia of applied ethics*, 2nd edn. San Diego: Academic Press.

H. ten Have (ed.) 2016. *Encyclopedia of Global Bioethics*. New York: Springer.

H. LaFollette (ed.) 2013. *International Encyclopedia of Ethics*. Oxford: Wiley-Blackwell.

Two excellent peer-reviewed online and open-access encyclopaedias are:

Internet Encyclopaedia of Philosophy (IEP): http://www.iep.utm.edu/
Stanford Encyclopaedia of Philosophy (SEP): https://plato.stanford. edu/

Three contrasting types of ethical theory are worth exploring: duty-based theories, utilitarianism, and virtue ethics.

Three chapters by Onora O'Neill (pp. 175–85), Nancy Davis (pp. 205–18), and Jonathan Dancy (pp. 219–29) in *A Companion to Ethics* edited by Peter Singer (Oxford: Blackwells) provide clear and fairly detailed accounts of various duty-based approaches to ethics:

For a short but rigorous account of Kant's moral theory, see:

R. Walker 1998. *Kant and the Moral Law*. London: Phoenix Orion Publishing Group, pp. 39–42; or

R. Scruton 2001. *Kant: A Very Short Introduction*. Oxford: Oxford University Press.

With regards to utilitarianism, key essays by its founders, Jeremy Bentham and John Stuart Mill can be found in:

Ryan (ed.) 1987. *Utilitarianism and other Essays: JS Mill and J Bentham*. Penguin: Harmondsworth.

A clear and wide-ranging book that provides a useful philosophical analysis of utilitarianism is:

R. Crisp 1997. *Mill on Utilitarianism*. London: Routledge.

Many modern medical ethicists, and also healthcare professionals, find the approach of 'virtue ethics' useful and interesting. A book that collects together several articles using a virtue ethics approach, some of which are in the field of medical ethics is:

R. Crisp and M. Slote (eds) 1997. *Virtue Ethics* (Oxford Readings in Philosophy). Oxford: Oxford University Press.

For a much larger textbook of medical ethics built around the pioneering 'four principle' approach to medical ethics analysis, see:

T.L. Beauchamp and J.F. Childress 2013. *Principles of Biomedical Ethics*, 7th edn. New York: Oxford University Press.

Other general books in medical ethics include:

M. Parker and D. Dickenson 2010. *The Cambridge Medical Ethics Workbook*, 2nd edn. Cambridge: Cambridge University Press. This provides many cases taken from healthcare across several European countries together with analyses of the cases. A combination of textbook and case book.

R.E. Ashcroft, A. Dawson, H. Draper, and J. McMillan 2007. *Principles of Health Care Ethics*, 2nd edn. New York: John Wiley. This is a scholarly and detailed encyclopaedia of theories, principles, and common ethical issues that arise in healthcare.

Two textbooks that are aimed predominantly towards medical students and junior doctors are:

D. Wilkinson, J. Herring, and J. Savulescu (in press). *Medical Ethics and Law: The core curriculum*, 3rd edn. Amsterdam: Elsevier.

P. Davey, A. Rathmell, M. Dunn, C. Foster, and H. Salisbury 2016. *Medical Ethics, Law and Communication: At a glance*. New York: Wiley.

The academic world shares ideas through journals as much as through books. Many of the articles, although by no means all, are readily accessible to the interested lay reader.

The Journal of Medical Ethics aims at health professionals as much as at philosophers. It also has a good website: https://jme.bmj.com/

Clinical Ethics is also aimed at health professionals, and has a strongly empirical orientation: http://journals.sagepub.com/home/cet

The Hastings Center Report covers a wide range of practical medical ethics and policy-oriented articles: https://www.thehastingscenter. org/publications-resources/hastings-center-report/

Five other major international journals in medical ethics with a mainly philosophical perspective are: *Bioethics*, the *American Journal of Bioethics*, *The Kennedy Institute of Ethics Journal*, *Medicine, Health Care and Philosophy*, and the *Cambridge Quarterly of Healthcare Ethics*.

Additional bodies, within and outside governments, produce reports relevant to medical ethical issues. These often provide ethical frameworks or guidance to think through the issues at a policy level. One such body is the Nuffield Council on Bioethics in the UK, which has produced a wide range of medical ethics reports: http://nuffieldbioethics.org/ Another body was The Presidential Commission for the Study of Bioethical Issues, which was established in 2009, but disbanded under the Trump Administration in 2017. Its reports have been archived: https://bioethicsarchive.georgetown.edu/pcsbi/index.html

The *Journal of Applied Philosophy* and the *Journal of Practical Ethics* cover applied philosophy generally. This includes such areas as environmental ethics, criminology, business ethics, as well as topics in medical ethics.

Chapter 2: Assisted dying: good medical practice, or murder?

An excellent, readable, and philosophically sophisticated discussion on ethical issues at the end of life is provided in:

J. Glover 1977. *Causing Death and Saving Lives*. London: Penguin.

A useful book that covers a wide range of issues in medicine at the end of life is:

D.W. Brock 1993. *Life and Death: Philosophical Essays in Biomedical Ethics*. Cambridge: Cambridge University Press.

The following book opens up a wider discussion about the ethics of killing, and different individuals' roles in ending life. Specific chapters focus on euthanasia, termination of pregnancy, and infanticide:

J. McMahan 2002. *The Ethics of Killing: Problems at the Margins of Life*. Oxford: Oxford University Press.

If you want to read more about euthanasia and physician assisted suicide in particular then the following four books are a good way in to the literature:

M. Battin, R. Rhodes, and A. Silvers (eds) 1998. *Physician Assisted Suicide: Expanding the Debate*. New York: Routledge.

E. Jackson and J. Keown 2012. *Debating Euthanasia*. Oxford: Hart.

R. Huxtable 2013. *Euthanasia: All that Matters*. London: Hodder & Stoughton.

If you would like to see how arguments about the ethics of deciding whether or not to end the lives of critically ill children are made, and are related to actual clinical practice, an excellent contribution is:

D. Wilkinson 2013. *Death or Disability? The 'Carmentis Machine' and Decision-making for Critically Ill Children*. Oxford: Oxford University Press.

Chapter 3: A toolbox of reasoning

There is a wide range of resources that introduce philosophical techniques of argumentation and critical reasoning. A clear and thorough examination of thinking about how to think in ethics that is illustrated with many examples is:

A. Thomson 1999. *Critical Reasoning in Ethics*. London: Routledge.

A useful source book of types of fallacy and of valid reasoning in a simple dictionary style is:

N. Warburton 2007. *Thinking from A to Z*, 3rd edn. London: Routledge.

For an entertaining introduction to formal logic, see:

G. Priest 2000. *Logic: A Very Short Introduction*. Oxford: Oxford University Press. This book has a good account of the sorites paradox and the slippery slope argument, but, despite its brevity and accessibility, this book gets into some pretty technical stuff.

For a lively, but far from superficial, introduction to ethics, and ethical thinking, see:

S. Blackburn 2001. *Ethics: A Very Short Introduction*. Oxford: Oxford University Press.

And if you want to take a further step back—from ethics to philosophy more generally—see:

E. Craig 2002. *Philosophy: A Very Short Introduction*. Oxford: Oxford University Press.

The critical philosophical tradition—the tradition of argument—began in ancient Greece around the 6th century BC. An excellent introduction to Greek philosophy is:

J. Annas 2000. *Ancient Philosophy: A Very Short Introduction.* Oxford: Oxford University Press.

And why not dip into Plato himself, and meet Socrates as both questioner and orator. An engaging place to start is with the Plato dialogues that are sometimes brought together as the 'Trial and Death of Socrates': Euthyphro, Apology (an account of Socrates' trial, and one of the dramatic masterpieces of Western literature), Crito, and Phaedo (which ends with Socrates' last words as the paralysing effects of hemlock creep up his body). All four are available (together with a fifth dialogue) in:

Plato 2002. *Five Dialogues: Euthyphro, Apology, Crito, Meno, and Phaedo*, trans. G.M.A. Grube, 2nd edn. London: Hackett Publishing Company.

Chapter 4: People who don't exist; at least not yet

The first major exploration of the non-identity problem from a philosophical angle is in:

Parfit D. 1984. *Reasons and Persons* (chapter 16). Oxford University Press: Oxford.

Additional analysis of the implications of the non-identity problem for doctors is given in:

T. Hope and J. McMillan 2012. Physicians' duties and the non-identity problem. *American Journal of Bioethics*, 12(8): 21–9. A number of commentaries from medical ethicists accompany this article, responding to the claims made.

An early and lively discussion of issues raised by the possibility of selecting the characteristics of our children is given in:

J. Glover 1984. *What Sort of People Should There Be?* Harmondsworth: Pelican; and

J. Glover 2006. *Choosing Children: Genes, Disability, and Design.* Oxford: Oxford University Press.

For a more polarized debate:

J. Savulescu and G. Kahane 2009. The moral obligation to create children with the best chance of the best life. *Bioethics*, 23(5): 274–90.

Or, if you prefer something shorter and more provocative:

J. Savulescu 2001. Procreative beneficence: why we should select the best children. *Bioethics*, 15(5/6): 413–26; and

R. Sparrow 2010. Should human beings have sex? Sexual dimorphism and human enhancement. *American Journal of Bioethics*, 10(7): 3–12.

The following two books provide an examination of a wide range of issues associated with assisted reproduction and the new genetics with an extensive cover of the associated literature:

R. Deech and A. Smajdor 2007. *From IVF to Immortality: Controversy in the Era of Reproductive Technology*. Oxford: Oxford University Press.

S. Wilkinson 2010. *Choosing Tomorrow's Children: The Ethics of Selective Reproduction*. Oxford: Oxford University Press.

The most obvious area of reproductive medicine that raises important ethical concerns is that of abortion. A brief overview of some of the main positions on abortion is given in:

D. Wilkinson, J. Herring, and J. Savulescu in press, 2018. *Medical Ethics and Law: The Core Curriculum*, 3rd edn. Amsterdam: Elsevier.

Two articles that provide perspectives on the morality of abortion that get away from the focus on the moral status of the embryo are:

J.J. Thomson 1971. A defence of abortion. *Philosophy and Public Affairs*, 1(1). (Reprinted in P. Singer (ed.) 1986. *Applied Ethics*. Oxford: Oxford University Press.); and

R. Hursthouse 1991. Virtue theory and abortion. *Philosophy and Public Affairs*, 20: 223–46. (Reprinted in R. Crisp and M. Slote (eds) 1997. *Virtue Ethics*. Oxford: Oxford University Press, pp. 217–38).

Chapter 5: Inconsistencies about madness

An excellent edited collection covering a wide range of areas of ethics and mental illness is:

S. Bloch and S.A. Green 2009. *Psychiatric Ethics*, 4th edn. Oxford: Oxford University Press.

The 'anti-psychiatry' movement of the 1960s produced some trenchant and well-written critiques of the whole idea of mental illness and the coercive ways in which society treats the mentally ill. Two of the most influential such books were:

R.D. Laing 1990. *The Divided Self.* London: Penguin Books. (First published 1960.)

T. Szasz 1984. *The Myth of Mental Illness*, revised edn. New York: Harper Collins. (First published 1960.)

It is in the field of mental illness that philosophical issues about the concept and classification of disease have been most discussed. There is an interesting collection of papers in the *Journal of Medical Ethics* offering ethical analyses of these issues in psychiatry:

G. Szmukler 2014. When psychiatric diagnosis becomes an overworked tool. *Journal of Medical Ethics*, 40(8): 517–20.

M.D. Pickersgill 2014. Debating DSM-5: diagnosis and the sociology of critique. *Journal of Medical Ethics*, 40(8): 521–5.

F. Callard 2014. Psychiatric diagnosis: the indispensibility of ambivalence. *Journal of Medical Ethics*, 40(8): 526–30.

J.S. Blumenthal-Barby 2014. Psychiatry's new manual (DSM-5): ethical and conceptual dimensions. *Journal of Medical Ethics*, 40(8): 531–6.

N. Bingham and N. Banner 2014. The definition of mental disorder: evolving but dysfunctional? *Journal of Medical Ethics*, 40(8): 537–42.

A good starting point for the literature on the abuse of psychiatry for political purposes is:

P. Chodoff 2009. The abuse of psychiatry, in S. Bloch and S.A. Green (eds), *Psychiatric Ethics*, 4th edn. Oxford: Oxford University Press.

Although not discussed in this chapter, there are many ethical issues that arise from the practice of psychotherapy. These are discussed in some detail in:

J. Holmes and R. Lindley 1998. *The Values of Psychotherapy*, revised
   edn. London: Karnac Books.

Chapter 6: Helping the helper

A good summary of the varied ethical challenges that arise in the care
and treatment of people with dementia is offered in:

Nuffield Council on Bioethics 2009. *Dementia: Ethical Issues*.
   London: Nuffield Council on Bioethics.

More general analyses of the ethics of community, residential, and
long-term care are also available. The following contributions examine
the extent to which values and principles in medical ethics need to be
amended or refined when applied to long-term care:

G. Agich 2003. *Dependence and Autonomy in Old Age: An Ethical
   Framework for Long-term Care*. Cambridge: Cambridge University
   Press.
T. Hope and M. Dunn 2014. The ethics of long-term care practice: a
   global call to arms, in A. Akabayashi (ed.), *The Future of Bioethics:
   International Dialogues*. Oxford: Oxford University Press.

Those writing about the ethics of long-term care have often drawn
on, and developed, a moral theory that emphasizes the moral
significance of care in itself. Literature on the 'ethics of care',
which is closely related to virtue ethics, is wide-ranging. Good
introductions include:

R. Tong 1998. The ethics of care: a feminist virtue ethics of care for
   healthcare practitioners. *Journal of Medicine and Philosophy*,
   23(2): 131–52.
V. Held 2005. *The Ethics of Care: Personal, Political, and Global*.
   Oxford: Oxford University Press.
J.C. Tronto 2014. Care ethics. *The Encyclopaedia of Political Thought*.
   Oxford: Wiley-Blackwell, pp. 442–3.

The cognitive changes characterized by the onset of dementia raise
questions about personhood. A good summary of these issues is
provided in the following report commissioned by Alzheimer Europe:

Alzheimer Europe 2013. *Personhood*. https://www.alzheimer-europe.
   org/Ethics/Definitions-and-approaches/Other-ethical-principles/
   Personhood

Connected to questions of personhood are questions about how the interests of the person with dementia should be conceptualized. A brief summary of the arguments about how to understand the interests of people with dementia can be found in:

Nuffield Council on Bioethics 2009. *Dementia: Ethical Issues*. London: Nuffield Council on Bioethics, ch. 5.

An important argument and counter-argument central to this debate is:

R. Dworkin 1993. *Life's Dominion: An Argument about Abortion, Euthanasia, and Individual Freedom*. New York: Knopf, see ch. 7.

R. Dresser 1995. Dworkin on dementia: elegant theory, questionable policy. *Hastings Center Report*, 25(6): 32–8.

Chapter 7: Establishing fair procedure

A defence of the particular procedural approach to ensure fairness in resource allocation decision-making described in this chapter is provided by Norman Daniels and James Sabin:

N. Daniels and J.E. Sabin 1997. Limits to health care: fair procedures, democratic deliberation, and the legitimacy problem for insurers. *Philosophy and Public Affairs*, 26: 303–50; and

N. Daniels and J.E. Sabin 2008. Accountability for reasonableness: an update. *BMJ*, 337: a1850.

This approach is strongly influenced by the more general approach to justice developed by John Rawls:

J. Rawls 1971. *A Theory of Justice*. Cambridge, MA: Harvard University Press.

A well-known and more libertarian approach to theorizing justice is offered by Nozick. This is the book that also introduces the Experience Machine thought experiment (see Chapter 3):

R. Nozick 1974. *Anarchy, State, and Utopia*. New York: Basic Books.

Another well-known position on justice against Rawls and Nozick is that offered by Cohen who defends a particular account of socialism:

G. Cohen 1995. *Self-Ownership, Freedom and Equality*. Cambridge: Cambridge University Press.

A comprehensive and very accessible summary of different theories of justice is offered in:

M. Sandel 2008. Justice: *What's the Right Thing to Do?* London: Penguin.

The argument against the 'rule of rescue' given in this chapter is based on:

T. Hope 2001. Rationing and life-saving treatment: should identifiable patients have higher priority? *Journal of Medical Ethics*, 27(3): 179–85.

Two other notable arguments against the rule of rescue are:

J. McKie and J. Richardson 2003. The rule of rescue. *Social Science and Medicine*, 56(12): 2407–19.

M. Verweij 2015. How (not) to argue for the rule of rescue: claims of individuals versus group solidarity, in I.G. Cohen, N. Daniels, and N. Eyal (eds), *Identified versus Statistical Lives: An Interdisciplinary Perspective*. New York: Oxford University Press.

Two defences of particular accounts of the rule of rescue are offered in:

M. Sheehan 2007. Resources and the rule of rescue. *Journal of Applied Philosophy*, 24(4): 352–66.

T. Rulli and J. Millum 2016. Rescuing the duty to rescue. *Journal of Medical Ethics*, 42(4): 260–4.

For a good collection of both practical and theoretical papers covering a wide range of contemporary issues in healthcare rationing, see:

A. Coulter and C. Ham (eds) 2000. *The Global Challenge of Health Care Rationing*. Buckingham: Open University Press; and

M. Battin, R. Rhodes, and A. Silvers (eds) 2012. *Medicine and Social Justice: Essays on the Distribution of Health Care*. New York: Oxford University Press. This book provides perspectives from both sides of the Atlantic.

P.M. Rosoff 2017. *Drawing the Line: Healthcare Rationing and the Cutoff Problem*. New York: Oxford University Press. This book offers an analysis of rationing in the US healthcare context in ways that are sympathetic to models of universal healthcare.

The King's Fund undertakes detailed work on cost-effectiveness and health policy, and has produced a number of reports on this topic for the UK context. A useful introduction to resource allocation in the English context is available:

D. Buck and A. Dixon. 2013. *Improving the Allocation of Health Resources in England: How to Decide Who Gets What.* London: The King's Fund. https://www.kingsfund.org.uk/sites/default/files/field/field_publication_file/improving-the-allocation-of-health-resources-in-england-kingsfund-apr13.pdf

For a contribution that more directly articulates a set of ethical principles for resource allocation in the UK, see:

M. Sheehan and T. Hope 2012. Allocating health care resources in the UK: putting principles into practice, in M. Battin, R. Rhodes, and A. Silvers (eds) 2012. *Medicine and Social Justice: Essays on the Distribution of Health Care.* New York: Oxford University Press, ch. 17.

Chapter 8: How modern genetics is testing traditional confidentiality

The ethical issues that arise from genetics and other new biotechnologies are the current growth industries of medical ethics. An excellent book on ethics and genetics is:

A. Buchanan, D.W. Brock, N. Daniels, and D. Wikler 2000. *From Chance to Choice: Genetics and Justice.* Cambridge: Cambridge University Press.

We also recommend two recent reports produced by the Nuffield Council on Bioethics which outline the ethical issues raised by a variety of new biotechnologies:

Nuffield Council on Bioethics 2012. *Emerging Biotechnologies: Teachnology, Choice and the Public Good.* London: Nuffield Council on Bioethics. http://nuffieldbioethics.org/project/emerging-biotechnologies

Nuffield Council on Bioethics 2013. *Novel Neurotechnologies: Intervening in the Brain.* London: Nuffield Council on Bioethics. http://nuffieldbioethics.org/project/neurotechnology

Perhaps the most famous case against the use of genetic engineering can be found in:

M.J. Sandel 2007. *The Case against Perfection*. Cambridge, MA: Harvard University Press.

Alternative ethical critiques of the potential of new biotechnologies relate to concerns about eugenics. The first book provides a good history of eugenics, and the second paper examines eugenics in relation to new technological developments:

D.J. Kevles 1995. *In the Name of Eugenics: Genetics and the Uses of Human Heredity*. Cambridge, MA: Harvard University Press.
D. Wikler 1999. Can we learn from eugenics? *Journal of Medical Ethics*, 25(2): 183–94.

Other commentators take issue with the discriminatory impact that advances in genetic technologies will have on the lives of people with disabilities. For a collection of papers on this point, see:

E. Parens and A. Asch (eds) 2000. *Prenatal Testing and Disability Rights*. Washington, DC: Georgetown University Press; and
E. Parens and A. Asch 2003. Disability rights critique of prenatal genetic testing: reflections and recommendations. *Mental Retardation and Developmental Disabilities Research Reviews*, 9(1): 40–7.

The Nuffield Council on Bioethics offers an updated analysis of the ethics of prenatal testing as new non-invasive methods for obtaining information about the genetic makeup of a foetus have become available:

Nuffield Council on Bioethics 2017. *Non-invasive Prenatal Testing: Ethical Issues*. London: Nuffield Council on Bioethics.

For a broader analysis of how genetics has become integrated into day to day medical practice, and the ethical issues that arise for those working in clinical genetics services, see:

M. Parker 2012. *Ethical Problems and Genetics Practice*. Cambridge: Cambridge University Press.

Chapter 9: Culture, consent, and community

Chapter 9 draws attention to a longstanding debate within medical ethics: whether the ethical principles that we articulated in Chapter 3 are universal, or whether they are relevant only to 'Western' healthcare settings. Many of these arguments have been made in considering whether there is a relevant difference between 'Western' and 'Asian' ethical theories, values, or principles. To delve into the arguments in this debate, see on the one hand:

H. Widdows 2007. Is global ethics moral neo-colonialism? An investigation of the issue in the context of bioethics. *Bioethics*, 21(6): 305–15.

H. Widdows 2011. Western and Eastern principles and globalised bioethics. *Asian Bioethics Review*, 3(1): 14–22; and on the other hand:

S. Chattopadhyay and R. de Vries 2008. Bioethical concerns are global, bioethics is western. *Eubios: Journal of Asian and International Bioethics*, 18(4): 106–9.

For a more recent example of these arguments, made in the context of multiculturalism, see:

C. Durante in press, 2018. Bioethics and multiculturalism: nuancing the discussion. *Journal of Medical Ethics*; and a response:

T.L. Beauchamp 2018. Comments on Durante's account of multiculturalism. *Journal of Medical Ethics*, 44(2): 84–5.

The position that we defended in this chapter is one that stresses the importance of cross-cultural argumentation. For a good example of this approach, see:

A. Akabayashi (ed.) 2014. *The Future of Bioethics: International Dialogues*. Oxford: Oxford University Press.

For an analysis of the specific steps that medical ethicists might undertake to establish dialogue and engagement with community members in different global contexts, try:

V.M. Marsh, D.M. Kamuya, A.M. Mlamba, T.N. Williams, and S.S. Molyneux 2010. Experiences with community engagement and informed consent in a genetic cohort study of severe childhood diseases in Kenya. *BMC Medical Ethics*, 11: 13.

P.Y. Cheah, K.M. Lwin, L. Phaiphun, L. Maelankiri, M. Parker, N.P. Day, N.J. White, and F. Nosten 2010. Community engagement on the Thai-Burmese border: rationale, experience and lessons learnt. *International Health*, 2(2): 123–9.

A point we explored in the chapter was that undertaking medical research in non-Western settings poses challenges to how research should be conducted. International guidelines try to harmonize medical research by addressing these ethical challenges. The two leading and most recent sets of guidelines for international research ethics are:

The Council for International Organizations of Medical Sciences 2016. *International Ethical Guidelines for Health-related Research Involving Humans*. Geneva: CIOMS.

World Medical Association 2013. *Declaration of Helsinki: Ethical principles for medical research involving human subjects*. Ferney-Voltaire: WMA.

A more academic report that provides an excellent and comprehensive overview of this issue is:

Nuffield Council on Bioethics 2002. *The Ethics of Research Related to Healthcare in Developing Countries*. London: Nuffield Council on Bioethics. http://nuffieldbioethics.org/project/research-developing-countries/

Including a follow up paper that examines these issues in relation to updated guidelines:

Nuffield Council on Bioethics 2005. *The Ethics of Research Related to Healthcare in Developing Countries: A Follow Up Paper*. London: Nuffield Council on Bioethics. http://nuffieldbioethics.org/project/research-developing-countries-follow

Chapter 10: A glance into the future

Our glance into the future suggested that ethicists are now spending considerable effort in exploring ethical issues related to scientific and technological advancements in medicine, which are either in development or have the potential for future clinical application.

Methods based on genetic or pharmacological advances could potentially be used, not to prevent disease or disability, but also to *enhance* human beings—for example to increase intelligence, or to increase a person's capacity to act morally. Most of us believe it is right to enhance children's intellectual abilities through good education. Is it right to enhance children's intelligence through gene therapy? For arguments generally in favour of various enhancement technologies, try:

N. Agar 2004. *Liberal Eugenics: In Defence of Human Enhancement.* Oxford: Blackwell.

J. Harris 2007. *Enhancing Evolution: The Ethical Case for Making Better People.* Princeton, NJ: Princeton University Press.

N. Bostrom and T. Ord 2006. The reversal test: eliminating status quo bias in applied ethics. *Ethics*, 116(4): 656–79.

A. Buchanan 2008. Enhancement and the ethics of development. *Kennedy Institute of Ethics Journal*, 18(1): 1–34.

A. Buchanan 2011. *Beyond Humanity? The Ethics of Biomedical Enhancement.* Oxford: Oxford University Press.

For responses to some of the arguments developed in these books and articles, see:

R. Sparrow 2011. A not-so-new eugenics, *The Hastings Center Report*, 41(1): 32–42.

M. Sandel 2004. The case against perfection: what's wrong with designer children, bionic athletes, and genetic engineering? *The Atlantic Monthly*, 292(3): 51–62.

For a comprehensive summary of the current debate, try:

J. Savulescu and N. Bostrom 2010. *Human Enhancement.* Oxford: Oxford University Press.

Or, for a shorter summary, the entry on:

T. Douglas 2013. Biomedical enhancement, in H. LaFollette (ed.), *International Encyclopedia of Ethics*. Oxford: Wiley-Blackwell.

In the last ten years, genome editing has emerged, and, in the past couple of years, a specific genome editing method, known as CRISPR-Cas 9 has begun to be used extensively in scientific research. This technique has a wide range of potential applications in medicine, agriculture, and industry. Genome editing involves altering a selected DNA sequence in a living cell, affecting how a gene functions. For a comprehensive summary of the ethical issues associated with future applications of this technology, see:

Nuffield Council on Bioethics 2016. *Genome Editing: An Ethical Review*. London: Nuffield Council on Bioethics; and

National Academy of Sciences, Engineering and Medicine 2017. *Human Genome Editing: Science, Ethics, and Governance*. Washington, DC: The National Academies Press.

For the argument in favour of gene editing, see:

C. Gyngell, T. Douglas, and J. Savulescu 2016. The ethics of germline gene editing. *Journal of Applied Philosophy*. https://doi.org/10.1111/japp.12249

Stem cell research has the potential, which is being rapidly realized, of developing novel and effective treatments. Carrying out such research raises ethical issues. See, for example:

K. Devolder 2015. *The Ethics of Embryonic Stem Cell Research*. Oxford: Oxford University Press.

Isolated human organs might be created from a person's cells (for example from a person's cheek cells) without creating a human being. Such organs could be immensely valuable in organ transplantation. It will soon be possible for human beings to be created from two parents of the same sex, or even from the cells of one 'parent'. It may also become possible to create novel creatures that combine human and animal parts. For discussions of the ethics of such possibilities, see:

T. Douglas, C. Harding, H. Bourne, and J. Savulescu 2012. Stem cell research and same-sex reproduction, in M. Quigley, S. Chan, and J. Harris (eds), *Stem Cells: New Frontiers in Science and Ethics*. London: World Scientific.

R. Streiffer 2010. Chimeras, moral status, and public policy: implications of the abortion debate for public policy on human/nonhuman chimera research. *The Journal of Law, Medicine & Ethics*, 38: 238–50.

R. Sparrow 2014. In vitro eugenics. *Journal of Medical Ethics*, 40: 725–31.

Synthentic biology involves creating artificial biological systems, with applications including synthetic DNA or a biological computer system.

Ethical concerns relate to the harms and benefits of these new applications, as well as questioning the changing relationship between human beings, the natural world and science. An extensive ethical analysis is provided in:

G.E. Kaebnick and T.H. Murray 2013. *Synthetic Biology and Morality: Artificial Life and the Bounds of Nature*. Cambridge, MA: MIT Press.

Finally, recent improvements to computing power and AI have numerous potential applications in the healthcare context. The analysis of big data sets to bring together a vast range of information about people's health experiences and personal backgrounds. Do patients have claims over these datasets, and how should the data be handled appropriately within a health system? The evolution of 'deep learning' techniques also means that doctors are becoming able to hand over decision-making about a person's health to a computer algorithm in order to improve diagnosis and treatment management.

A useful introduction to the ethics of big data in healthcare is provided in:

B.D. Mittelstadt and L. Floridi (eds) 2016. *The Ethics of Biomedical Big Data*. Dordrecht: Springer.

For an ethical debate about the wider scientific and medical application of AI, see:

S. Russell, S. Hauert, R. Altman, and M. Veloso 2015. Robotics: ethics of artificial intelligence. *Nature*, 521: 415–18.

For a more specific ethical analysis of algorithms in healthcare and other settings, see:

B.D. Mittelstadt, P. Allo, M. Taddeo, S. Wachter, and L. Floridi 2016. The ethics of algorithms: mapping the debate. *Big Data and Society*, 3: 1–21.

Index

Medical Ethics